Is Your Home Harming You?

How To Identify and Prevent Health Issues in Your Home

H.E. Rubin, M.S., M.P.H., M.S., Ph.D.

DEDICATION

To my beloved wife, Rimon, whose unwavering support and freedom have allowed me to pursue my passions, even in the face of uncertainty. Your care and dedication have been my guiding light.

To my children, Kay, Lisa, Sandy, and Joey, who have embraced my quirks with humor and curiosity. You are the only ones who could find joy in visits to garbage dumps, landfills, and wastewater treatment plants alongside your father.

And to my grandchildren, Lilly, Danny, Emily, Jasper, Pistachio, and those yet to come, I dedicate this book to you. May you grow up in a safer world, and may you carry forward the legacy of striving to make our planet a better place.

ACKNOWLEDGMENTS

I would like to acknowledge the help I received from my granddaughter, Lilly Reich, for her support throughout this project and her assistance in conducting research on various topics. Not only was she an asset, but I also enjoyed every minute we worked together.

Many people played important roles in the development of this book. I wish to thank Rachael Davidson for her guidance, insights, and help in processing my thoughts. We had many interesting conversations together. Next, I would like to thank Walter Haskins for ensuring that the book's development progressed properly. I also want to thank Garryson Johnson for his contributions to the book's development. Finally, I would like to thank James Marshal for creating the book cover and the logo, Max Parker for the graphics, and Dexter Owens for the marketing. Without their help, this project may never have come to fruition.

Lastly, I wish to acknowledge the hundreds of people who allowed me access to determine if their homes contained hazardous substances. Through my investigations and discussions with the residents, I gained a greater understanding of the health-related issues resulting from toxic household exposures. Sadly, many of these individuals died due to their exposures. I knew many of them well and considered them friends. I am honored to have known them. In their last hours, they wanted to help prevent this from happening to others, which speaks volumes about their character.

ABOUT THE AUTHOR

Dr. Rubin was born in the Bronx and lived in New York until he was 12 years old, when his family moved to rural North Carolina. After completing high school, he graduated with a BS in Biology from Guilford College. He received an MS in Medical Microbiology from Wake Forest University's School of Medicine, and from the University of Michigan's School of Public Health, he obtained an MPH in Water Quality, an MS in Food Science, and a Ph.D. in Environmental Health Science.

After graduation from the University of Michigan, Dr. Rubin worked as a consultant for the United States Agency for International Development (USAID) in Brazil. He then worked for a food manufacturing company, where he created their food testing laboratory and established QA/QC standards. Dr. Rubin was an NIH Postdoctoral Fellow at Cornell University, where he studied the biodegradation of man-made chemicals in freshwater. As a professor of microbiology at Rutgers University, he conducted research in the field of microbial ecology.

Dr. Rubin spent over 20 years in the environmental field as an environmental health scientist, working for environmental consulting firms and the New Jersey Department of Environmental Protection. At the New Jersey Department of Health, he served as an environmental toxicologist, overseeing field investigations of hazardous waste sites, risk assessments, data analyses, remediation feasibility studies, environmental mitigation, and toxicological analyses of human exposures to hazardous materials. His specialties include human and environmental exposure to hazardous waste and environmental toxicology. As an adjunct professor, he teaches courses in medical microbiology to nursing students, as well as courses in environmental science, environmental health, public health, biology, anatomy and physiology, and toxicology.

CONTENTS

CHAPTER 1: HIDDEN DANGERS AT HOME

There has been an increase in the number of television commercials promoting "green" products that are "good" for the environment. Several initiatives have been taken toward a healthy environment. Concerned not-for-profit institutions are raising environmental awareness in society. Sustainable activities are endorsed by schools to adopt responsible environmental habits. Thus, the general public is becoming aware of environmental problems and their consequences. These are just a few examples of the everyday exposures that people are subjected to regarding the hazards our activities pose to the environment and, consequently, to ourselves.

While outdoor pollution and its hazards are hot topics these days, virtually no attention is being given to our indoor environment. Pollution is not just restricted to oil spills at sea, increasing amounts of plastic waste, or the improper disposal of agricultural waste into natural bodies of water. Pollution is not so "singular," and it consists of any activity that can introduce harmful substances into an environment.

The environment can be considered to be the surroundings in which a person lives. It can be big or small. It can stretch out to faraway deserts and rainforests on the other side of the world, or it can be your basement or the next-door room in your home, within your confined vicinity. Therefore, it is even more important to control pollution in your homes and alleviate pollution from your personal dwellings than our outdoor environment because we spend the bulk of our time living indoors.

Often, people who have a general malaise will see a physician to determine the cause of their malaise, only to be told to adopt a healthier lifestyle. However, lifestyle changes do not always result in an improvement in health. So, they do research on their symptoms, but there are no conclusive results. It is frustrating because there is no visible manifestation.

They finally go on a vacation to relax. Surprisingly, they start to feel much better as the symptoms vanish. While remaining at home, you have symptoms. When you go outside for a period of time, the symptoms dissipate. This indicates that the cause of the symptoms may emanate from the home. Therefore, the house must contain a pollutant that poses a threat to your health. Everyone assumes that their house is a place in which they can be safe. It is quite natural to think this way.

This assumption can partially be attributed to the idea that we are the stakeholders in our places. By regularly cleaning our houses and being hygienic, we assume that there will be no household health-related problems. Thus, it is widely believed that there are environmental dangers outside our homes, but environmental problems are not associated with the home. Unfortunately, this is not the case. The interiors of homes usually pose greater threats to our health than when we are outside. The difference is that environmental problems inside our homes are less obvious to us. Household problems usually cause an extremely slow-paced decline in our health. The decline in our health is so subtle that it is not recognizable. The purpose of this book is to bring your attention to the threats in and around your home and how to mitigate them. Let us now explore how our homes contribute to a buildup of indoor pollutants, leading to significant yet undetected health impacts.

The first thought that may come to mind when the term air pollution pops up is probably carbon emissions or industrial waste. However, there are other contributors as well. The Environmental Protection Agency (EPA) of the USA claims that indoor air is two to five times more polluted than outdoor air. A plethora of factors can be held responsible, ranging from Volatile Organic Compounds (VOCs) emitted by some plants to more serious issues like the presence of radioactive substances. Harmful gases emitted by kitchen stoves, packaged spray products, household appliances like refrigerators and air conditioners, and direct or passive smoking through cigarettes, hookahs, and vapes are a few examples of other sources of indoor air pollution.

The symptoms resulting from the adverse health effects caused by living in a poor air-quality environment may not be apparent for years due to long-term, prolonged exposure. This may be one of the causes behind the increasing prevalence of diseases like asthma, humidifier fever, and pneumonitis. In addition to such long-term effects, short-term reactions like allergies, runny noses and eyes, and throat irritation may also occur. A simple cough may be a marker for a more severe, fulminating disease. Controlling this type of pollution is relatively simple because all that needs to be done is identify the sources of pollution and then eliminate them.

Formaldehyde, chlorofluorocarbons, benzene, naphthalene, methane, and carbon monoxide are some of the toxic gases that are commonly found in the home. They are usually colorless, odorless, and tasteless, which means that you probably are not aware of their presence in your home. If you are reading this indoors, there is a good chance that you are inhaling at least one of these gases as we speak. Many of the products we use in our daily routines emit these chemicals. Old bags and shoes may have started to decompose, discharging toxic chemicals like dioxins and furans. Similarly, the glue used to set PVC flooring in place can be hydrolyzed to produce phthalates, butylbenzene, and other contaminants.

The hazards of radioactive substances are now common knowledge, and they may be found in the home. The most common domestic radioactive element is Radon-222, a breakdown product of uranium, which is ubiquitous in nature. Radiation can cause genetic damage, resulting in various types of cancer and autoimmune diseases. The onset of cancer is usually asymptomatic, meaning it creates no symptoms until it is actively growing and causing organ damage.

Radon-222 and Radon-226 can be found in the soil and rocks on which our homes are built. It can enter a home through cracks and crevices in the foundation, seeping into low-level rooms where it may remain. According to the EPA, Radon alone is responsible for about 14,000 deaths per year in the United States. Therefore, great caution must be taken when choosing the site for building your house.

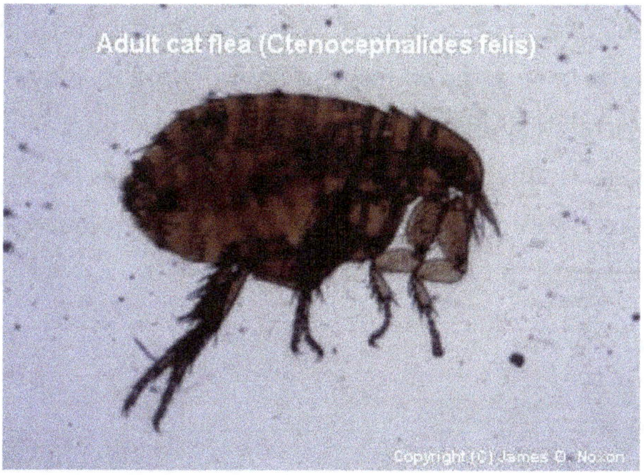

There are animals that share our house, such as rodents, fleas, bed bugs, dust mites, mildew, and fungus. These creatures can be annoying, in addition to the health risks they pose. Controlling them requires your active participation. Routinely cleaning the house and changing the bedding are important ways to lessen the intensity of these infestations.

Electromagnetic radiation (EMF) in the home comes from wires carrying electrical currents. Short-term exposure can occur when you are near electric appliances such as microwaves, refrigerators, washing machines, and televisions. This exposure can cause headaches, fatigue, stress, sleep disturbances, and skin symptoms such as rashes, prickling and burning sensations, and muscle aches. There is some evidence that it may also cause cancer. Therefore, we should be aware of this potential hazard.

Accidents are the fourth leading cause of death in the United States, after heart attacks, cancer, and strokes. However, about 78% of preventable injury-related deaths from unintentional accidents occur at home. Therefore, we should be cognizant of the causes of accidents and how to prevent them. Home is the place you turn to after an intense day of work or play. It should be comfortable and free from danger—your port in a storm. Thus, you must ensure that your home is as safe as possible. Read on to discover in detail the threats to your sanctuary regarding safety and ways to handle them.

CHAPTER 2: UNDERSTANDING HOUSEHOLD TOXINS

Science has its own vocabulary. Therefore, this chapter is devoted to explaining the most important terms that will be used to better understand the information. This will help you navigate through the book more smoothly and give you a better understanding of the content presented.

The first pair of words to be introduced are **toxic** and **hazardous**. Often, they are used interchangeably, but they have distinct meanings. **Hazardous** is an umbrella term that refers to the potential of a substance to cause harm to people, property, or the environment. There are seven hazardous categories: explosives, flammable liquids and solids, oxidizing substances, gases that are toxic or flammable, corrosive substances, toxic substances, and radioactive materials. The potential for harm can result directly from the substance, such as its physical or chemical properties, or indirectly from its potential to react with other substances.

Toxicity refers to the ability of a substance to cause harm to living organisms if it comes into contact with or enters the body. Exposure to a toxic substance can cause illness, injury, or even death. Thus, any poisonous chemical is considered a toxic substance. The term **hazardous** is general and all-encompassing; therefore, toxicity is just one of the classifications that can be used to describe a hazardous substance.

The term **ignitable** is used to describe a substance that can easily catch fire or burn, such as nail polish removers or hand sanitizers. **Corrosive** materials are those that gradually deteriorate or react with a material they are in direct contact with, typically metals or living tissues. This is the case for acids or lye. **Explosive** is a self-explanatory term for objects that can cause an explosion. Lastly, **reactive** substances can vigorously or even violently give off heat when they come in contact with air, water, or other common substances. Any substance that exhibits any of these properties is considered hazardous and should be avoided and handled with care.

Pay attention to **biohazard** signs. These signs indicate very dangerous materials, and therefore, they should not be taken lightly. If you see a container with this label, do not touch it. It may or may not be dangerous, but why take the chance? Remember that curiosity can kill the cat. On several occasions, I have seen people who did not respect the biohazard warning, and it never ended well for them.

Exposure to radioactive substances can cause chromosomal mutations, meaning it has the potential to irreversibly alter the genetic information of cells. These mutations can result in cancer-related teratogenic effects (birth defects) and a host of other conditions.

Radon, a disintegration product of radium, can be present in a home's atmosphere. It is a colorless, odorless, and tasteless gas; thus, the residents of the home would probably not be aware of its presence. Radon gas can decay into radioactive particles, which, when inhaled, can get trapped in the lungs. These particles release energy, which can damage lung tissue and result in lung cancer. Continuous exposure over time could lead to increasing fatigue, shortness of breath, a worsening cough, hoarseness, or trouble swallowing.

Radium

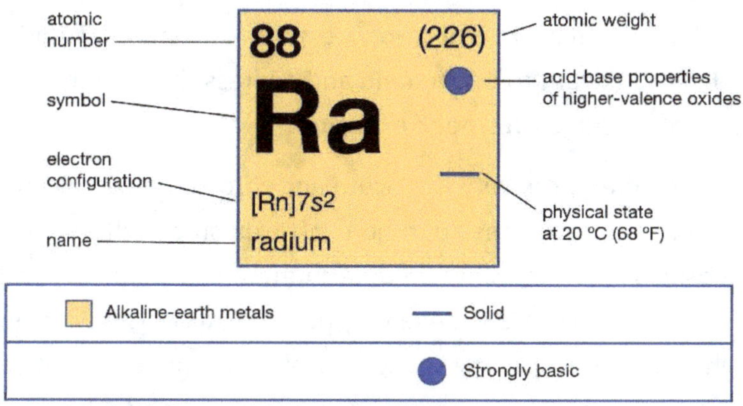

( ) indicates the mass of the longest-lived isotope.

There are two terms that refer to the duration of exposure to a toxic substance. **Acute exposure** is the term used to denote short-term exposure, whereas **chronic exposure** reflects long-term exposure. The United States Environmental Protection Agency (USEPA) considers exposure that is less than a year in length to be acute exposure. If a person's exposure is more than a year, it is considered chronic exposure.

Exposure to a toxic substance can occur for a few seconds, or it can last for minutes, hours, days, or even years. The symptoms resulting from acute exposures tend to emerge rapidly. For example, a person who is sensitized to pollen will have an allergic reaction whenever they are exposed to pollen. Conversely, chronic exposure can lead to a gradual decline in health. Since this decline is imperceptibly slow, the cause of the deterioration of a person's health may never be determined. Living in a house containing mold would result in continuous exposure, which could last for years. Every time a sensitive individual enters the house, they start sneezing. When they leave, there are no further problems. Both acute and chronic exposures warrant attention, and it's important to understand and address the potential risks associated with each type of exposure.

The differences between acute and chronic exposure can be greater than just the duration of exposure. Often, acute exposures result in the rapid deterioration of a person's health because the poison is either a very potent toxin or is present in a high concentration. This is why symptoms appear relatively quickly. Chronic exposure may involve exposure to less toxic substances or to very low concentrations of a toxicant for a long period of time.

Chronic exposure usually results in an insidious decline in an individual's health. It is often so slow that the person is not aware that their health is declining. If they do notice a decline in their health, they may attribute it to increasing age, a lack of sleep, or a poor lifestyle. Thus, they overlook the cause of the decline in their health. Many toxins can accumulate in the body over time. Continuous exposure may result in the gradual buildup of these substances in organs and tissues, leading to an increased risk of chronic diseases.

There are three ways in which a toxic substance can enter our bodies. I call them the **three I's of exposure**: inhalation, ingestion, and injection. Inhalation is the primary and most common method of exposure to harmful substances and pathogens in the home. Our body has protective mechanisms, including mucus covering the respiratory passages, the ciliary escalator, which removes particles and organisms from the respiratory passages, and lymphatic tissue, which can destroy pathogens. If a substance can pass these barriers, then it can cause damage. The longer the exposure, the greater its concentration, and the more potential damage can result. It's impossible to stop breathing, and wearing masks and face shields is of limited value. Thus, we are susceptible to inhaling particulates, volatile organic compounds (VOCs), viruses, bacteria, or fungi floating around in the atmosphere of the home.

The next "I" is ingestion, which refers to the consumption of food or water. If the food or water is tainted with chemicals or contains pathogens, then these will be ingested as well. Our body has relatively strong defenses; the stomach has a low pH, high acidity, and many enzymes that can destroy many toxins and pathogens. The intestines contain a complex community of microflora, which helps protect us from pathogenic microorganisms. Additionally, the immune system can play an important role in protecting us from pathogens and can help neutralize toxins.

Unfortunately, toxic substances are often water-soluble and can be quickly absorbed directly into the bloodstream. Despite our natural defenses, we are vulnerable to these silent killers and must implement habits that keep us out of harm's way.

Lastly, injection is another way that toxins and pathogens can enter our bodies. Injection can occur either through a laceration or cut in the skin or via penetration through the skin, such as by a snake bite or bee sting. Even a small wound can put us at risk. The risk factors are significantly elevated when organisms like molds, fungi, rodents, or mice inhabit the same space as you. Toxic substances may also enter your body via these portals of exposure.

In addition to the three portals of entry, a person can also be at risk through dermal contact. Some substances can irritate your skin, while others may be absorbed through the skin into the underlying tissues or into the circulatory system.

In conclusion, chronic exposure is of greater concern in households than acute exposure because it is more insidious and harder to determine. The concentration of a pollutant, its toxicity, the duration of exposure, its chemical properties, the portal of entry, the overall health of an individual, their lifestyle, their age, and many other factors influence the potency of a toxic substance. Understanding the cumulative effects, addressing multiple routes of exposure, and implementing preventive measures are essential for promoting a healthier indoor environment and minimizing the long-term health risks associated with chronic exposure to toxicants.

CHAPTER 3: BATTLING BIOLOGICAL THREATS

When addressing health hazards caused by our surroundings, biological threats are often overlooked. It is a common misassumption that once the dirt is removed, our houses are clean and safe. Unfortunately, however, that is not the case. We are cohabitating with a plethora of other organisms. You may be thinking that I am referring to mice and cockroaches. Perhaps you think that you have nothing to worry about because you do not leave food lying around. Unfortunately, there are other organisms to consider than just cockroaches and mice. These include rodents like rats and insects and even organisms that might not even be visible to the naked eye, such as mold, dust mites, mold, mildew, bacteria, and viruses. In this chapter, these organisms will be discussed along with the threats they pose and ways to eliminate them.

Rodents

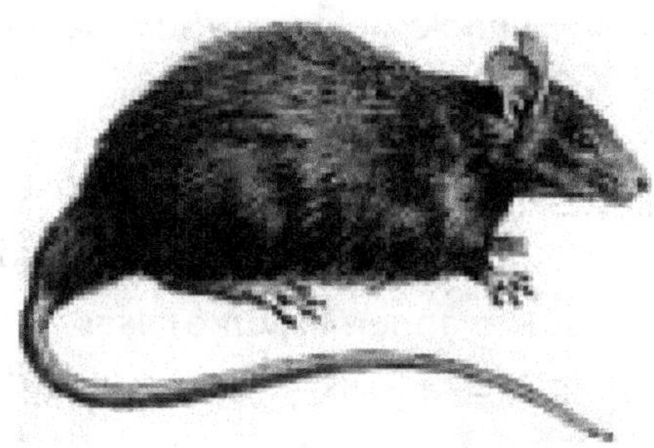

Rodents are harbingers of disease. They can transmit pathogenic bacteria and viruses directly through their bites, urine, and feces or indirectly by `contact with fleas. Ensure that you're not creating an environment conducive to rodents. If a rodent does make its way inside your house, take immediate action. The most common rodents are house mice and rats.

Usually, mice are timid and hide, while Norway rats can be very aggressive and even attack humans. There are documented cases where they have attacked adults and even bitten babies in their cribs.

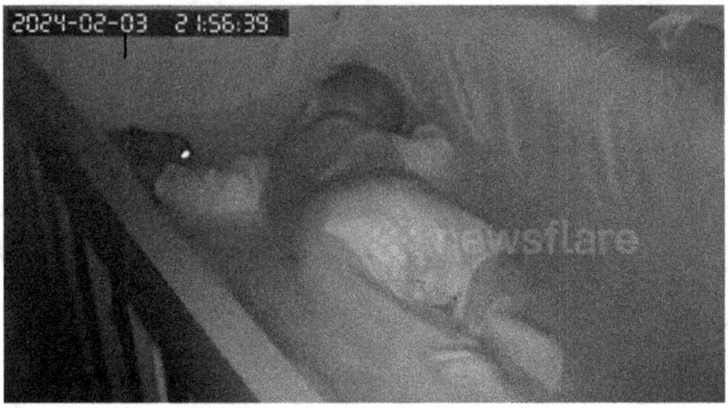

There are other species of rats, such as roof rats, that are relatively less aggressive and, as their name suggests, live on rooftops.

Rodents are nocturnal animals and are usually quite introverted. Thus, they are most active at night, preferring corners and other dark areas. Therefore, regularly clean crevices and corners, and keep an eye out for feces and dander. Today, many people delegate their cleaning responsibilities to various types of robots, making it hard to find evidence of rodents.

Another clue to their presence could be damaged foods and goods. Your clothes could have holes in them or be torn in an unusual manner. In some cases, rodents have gnawed at electric wires, leading to power outages. Female mice and rats can mature in two to three months and then have litters of offspring every two months. Thus, each female can produce 75 to 90 offspring per year. Multiply that by the baby female rates that are born, and you can have a massive infestation. This is why it is imperative to take action as soon as you see evidence of their presence.

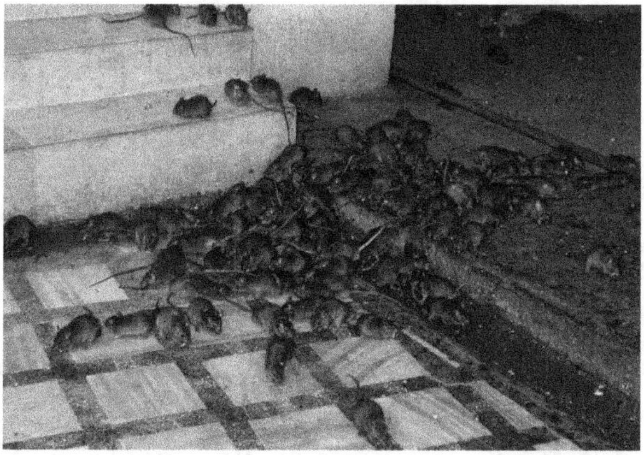

It is recommended that a deep cleaning of the house be done at least once a month. Rodents can cause various diseases like Rat-Bite Fever, Hemorrhagic Fever, Lassa Fever, Leptospirosis, Hantavirus Pulmonary Syndrome, Lymphocytic Choriomeningitis, Tularemia, Salmonellosis, and even Asthma. These are spread through the contamination of food or utensils. To illustrate, multiple deaths occurred in an area, and investigators found that it was due to a bacterial infection of *Leptospira,* which causes leptospirosis, commonly known as Weil's syndrome. It originated from contaminated soda cans in a warehouse that had dried rat urine on them.

Since rodents are attracted to the smell of food, make sure to store it properly. No scraps or other edible items should be left in the open. Leftovers should be stored in refrigerators and airtight containers that prevent their smell from wafting around.

Moreover, it quickly disposes of garbage, especially organic waste, as it decomposes and makes a scrumptious rodent meal.

Despite taking these precautions, there are various ways to get rid of them. Frequently, people use traps to catch rodents. There are physical traps that capture them alive by attracting them by using bait like cheese and peanut butter, which are quite effective. There are also traditional traps that, when activated, will snap shut, instantly breaking their necks. This is a humane way to exterminate rodents. However, these traps are not always successful, as rodents, especially rats, are quite intelligent and can figure out ways to steal the bait without tripping the trap. Place the traps in dark corners where it's most likely for the rodents to come into contact with them. You may choose to poison the food that eventually kills them. However, this is not recommended because they may die in an unreachable spot, like under furniture or behind walls. This is undesirable because of the smell that would be produced by their decomposing bodies and the insects that they might attract.

Insects

This brings us to the next fiend: insects. Although they may be small in size, they can be found in large numbers. The most common insect pest is cockroaches. They are nocturnal creatures that continuously look for leftovers. Even the little ones are exceptionally fast at getting out of sight when the lights are turned on. They are so commonplace that a certain number of insect parts are allowed in cereal. One aspect of cereal quality control consists of counting the number of insect parts.

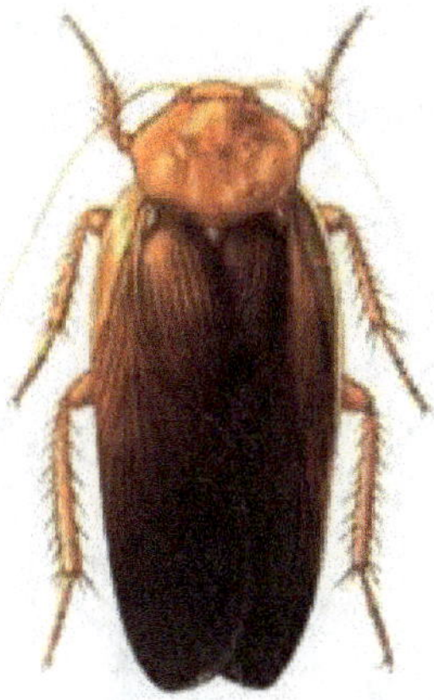

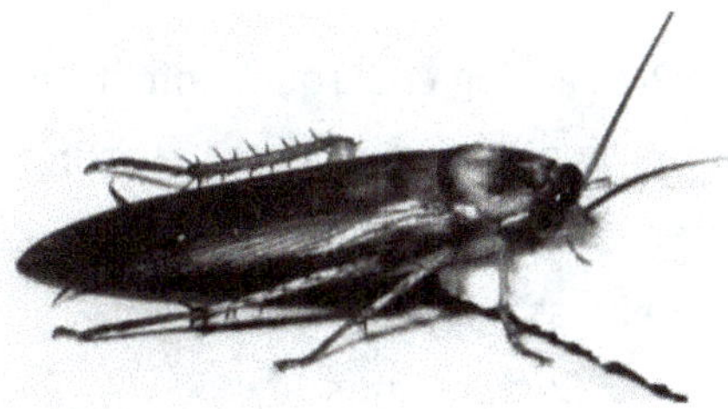

There are many different species of cockroaches, including Australian, Oriental, German, and brown-banded cockroaches. However, they are all potentially lethal. They can transmit 32 different bacterial, 17 fungal, 3 protozoan, and 2 viral diseases. The resulting diseases include Tuberculosis, Polio, Cholera, Leprosy, Dysentery, Typhoid, and various types of Gastroenteritis. Asthma may also result from the inhalation of cockroaches' feces or body parts. Transmission occurs by inhaling feces and either inhaling or ingesting body parts. Just like rodents, they will eat any organic matter they can detect. Due to their small size and their ability to compress themselves, they can easily enter the house. They can reproduce at an unprecedented rate. Cockroaches live for about a year, and in that time period, a female German cockroach can produce about 300,000 offspring. Of course, their offspring produce offspring as well, quickly resulting in an infestation. Therefore, the sooner you detect them, the easier it is to eradicate them. These infestations can become too large to contain. For example, in 2010, a house in Illinois was so severely infested by cockroaches that the authorities had no other option but to burn the place down.

Preventing cockroach infestations involves a combination of good hygiene practices, sealing entry points, and using deterrents.

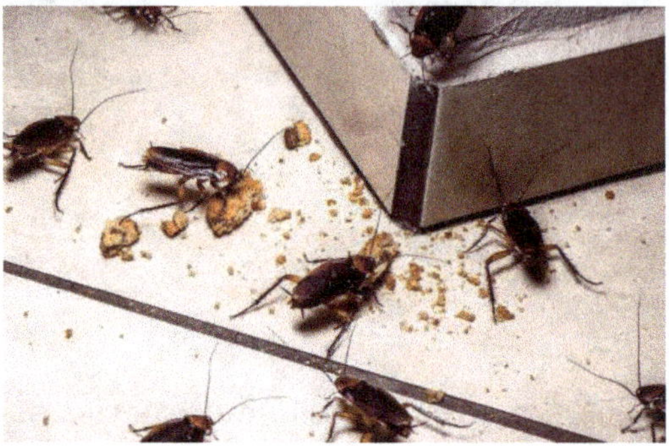

Cleanliness is the key. Cockroaches can be avoided by properly storing food and disposing of waste, just as rodent infestations can be prevented. Some natural substances, like peppermint oil, catnip, or bay leaves, are believed to repel cockroaches. You can place these around potential entry points or areas where cockroaches are seen. Boric acid is frequently used. However, it can pose a potential threat if consumed by pets and crawling infants. Diatomaceous earth is non-toxic and can be used to seal open cracks. This works by dehydrating and killing the insects.

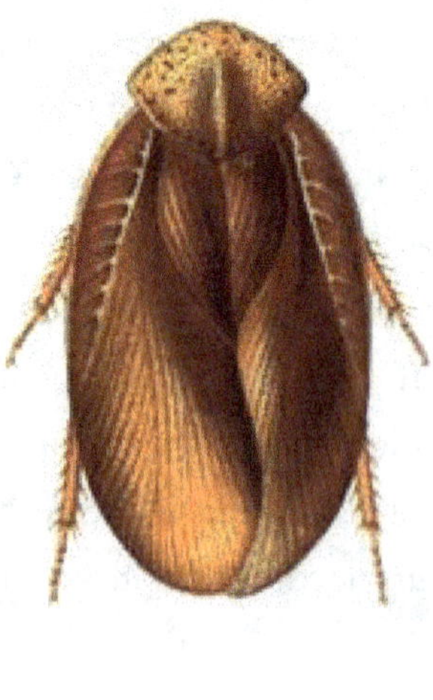

Dust mites are found in our pillows, comforters, carpets, and mattresses, but unfortunately, we cannot easily see them due to their small size. They can infest our bedding in large quantities. In fact, they can comprise about 10% of the weight of our bedding, thus making the bedding several pounds heavier. They feast on the dead cells we shed, and their feces can be covered with fungi due to their drool. While they don't directly cause severe illness, they can trigger allergic reactions, resulting in excessive sneezing, itching, a runny nose, and red eyes. These mites can attach to airborne particles, causing respiratory problems as well.

To minimize their adverse health effects, mattresses and pillows should be encased in covers, and bedding should be changed at least once a week. We cannot prevent them from invading our bedding, nor can we easily kill them. However, we can control our exposure to them by taking these precautions.

If you have pets in your house, you can be at risk of fleas, which they may carry in their fur. These tiny, wingless insects hop from one place to another and feed off mammalian blood. This should concern you, as these insects can also affect humans, putting you at risk of contracting infections from the pathogens they carry. Inside the house, they often live under carpets and in cracks and crevices like other insects. Huge global catastrophes like the bubonic plague and pneumonic plague can be attributed to these minuscule beings. Needless to say, they can be carried by rats.

Bed bugs are small, brownish-red, wingless insects. They dwell in beds and painlessly feed on humans while they are sleeping. They prefer to feed on the blood of humans but can also feed on other warm-blooded

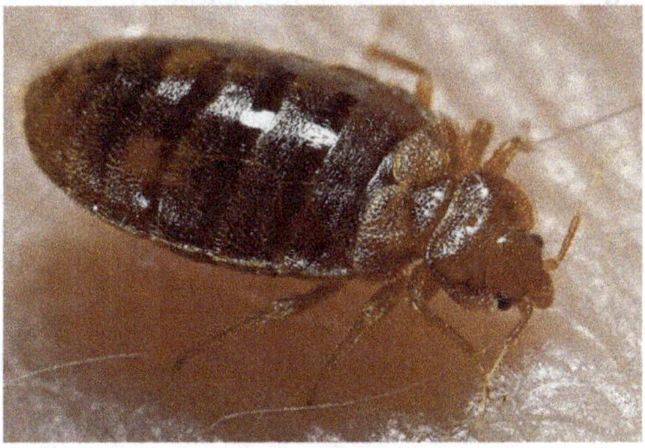

animals. It only takes five to ten minutes for them to engorge with blood. They are difficult to detect and can be transported from one place to another by latching onto suitcases, clothes, and linens. This is why bed bugs spread so easily. Females can lay one to five eggs per day, and it only takes 21 days for the nymphs to become adults.

Allergies can develop in the saliva that is transmitted during a bite, causing the area of the bite to become red, itchy, and swollen. Other symptoms are headache, dizziness, nausea,

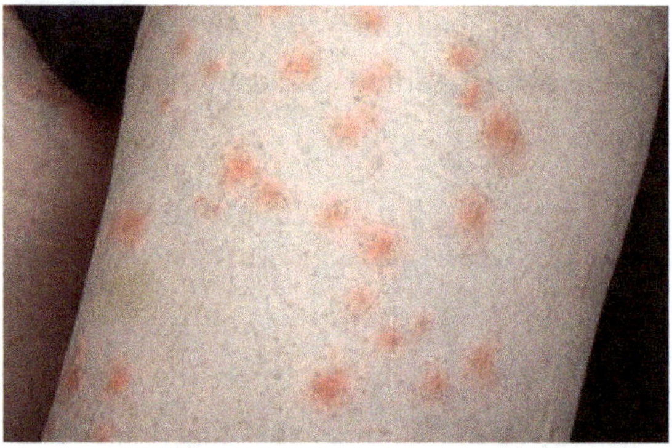

vomiting, diarrhea, fatigue, and increased salivation. They may cause secondary infections of the skin, resulting in impetigo, ecthyma, and lymphangitis. They may be able to transmit Staphylococcal infections, result in fungal diseases, carry the Trypanosome that causes Chagas disease, and transmit the pathogens that cause leprosy, brucellosis, and Q-fever. Bed bugs are definitely responsible for mental health problems.

Bed bugs can most easily be identified by small reddish-brown fecal spots that can be found on mattresses, upholstery, and walls or by bites on the arms and legs. Infestations can be confirmed by the observation of bed bug eggs, empty eggshells, and molt skins or by seeing the bugs themselves. To eliminate bed bugs, wash bedding, curtains, and clothing in hot water and dry them with high heat. Wash bedding regularly, and old ones should be discarded and replaced with fresh ones. Use a stiff brush to scrub mattress seams to remove bed bugs and their eggs before vacuuming. Be patient because it will take time to get rid of them.

Another potentially deadly insect is the mosquito, which, as we all know, also feeds on blood as its source of food. They have been found to cause Malaria, Yellow Fever, and Dengue fever. Other less common diseases include Eastern Equine Encephalitis, Western Equine Encephalitis, West Nile Encephalitis, St. Louis Encephalitis, Zika virus, and Chikungunya virus. They were also spread through mosquitoes. These illnesses can have severe consequences, ranging from flu-like symptoms to neurological complications and, in the case of the Zika virus, birth defects. It is evident that these insects are not to be taken lightly and definitely not to be allowed inside your house. Beyond the direct transmission of diseases, mosquito bites can cause extreme discomfort due to itching and severe allergic reactions in some individuals. Scratching mosquito bites can lead to secondary bacterial infections, further complicating the health risks associated with these insects.

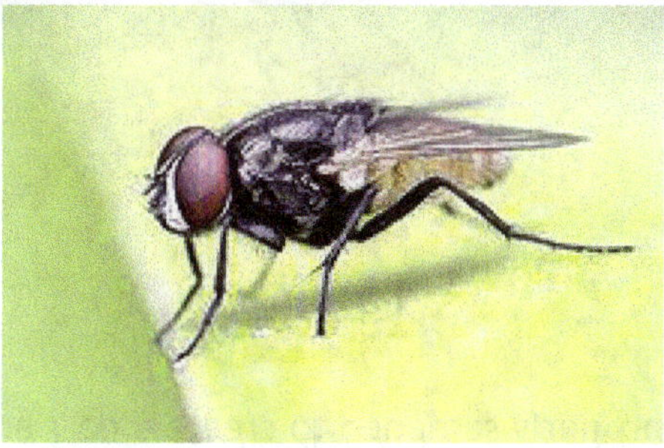

House flies are seemingly harmless creatures that can pose significant health risks because they can cause various diseases by picking up pathogenic microorganisms on their legs and mouths and then spreading them to surfaces or food. They can pick up bacteria and viruses from decaying organic matter, garbage, and feces and then transfer these microorganisms to food, kitchen surfaces, and utensils. Common diseases associated with house flies include gastroenteritis, cholera, dysentery, and respiratory infections.

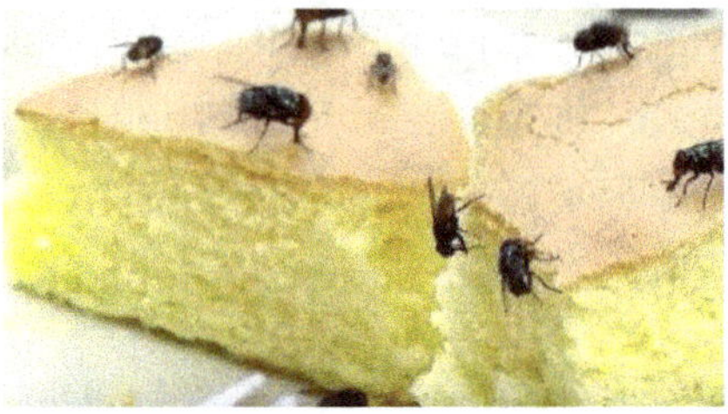

As always, the best time to act is when you first see any of these insects. The longer you wait, the worse the problem can become. A simple way to rid yourself of these bugs and the threats they pose is through the use of insecticide sprays. It works fast and is easy to apply, but insecticides may be toxic.

The best and most effective way to use insecticides is to spray the outside of the house to create a protective barrier that will prevent insects from entering. Try to avoid spraying indoors, as it can leave a chemical residue on the floor and furniture, which can be harmful if ingested by a toddler or pet.

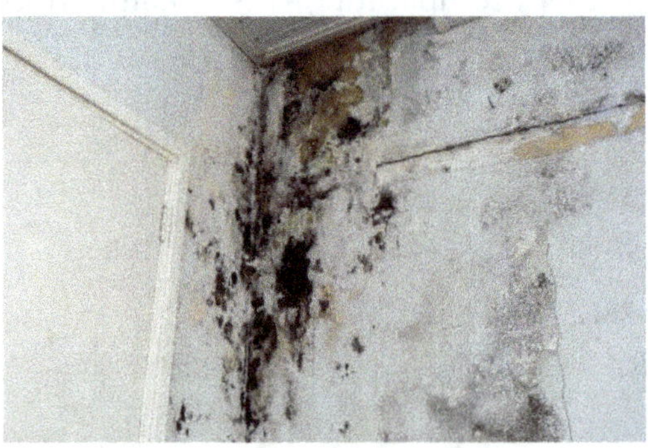

To control mosquitoes and other pests, remove any stagnant water that is around the house. Further, ensure that window and door screens are properly screened to create a barrier between flying insects and indoor living spaces. Vigilance is the key to controlling biological threats.

Mold and Mildew

Mildew and mold are types of fungi that thrive in damp and humid environments, making them common problems. Mildew is a type of mold that develops on damp surfaces such as walls, doors, shower grouting, windowsills, and anywhere that has high moisture levels. It appears as small, flat black spots and occasionally has a powdery texture. Mildew is frequently incorrectly used to refer to mold. Molds are microscopic fungi that grow via the production of multicellular filaments called hyphae. They encompass a much larger number of species than mildew. They can thrive on clothing, leather, paper, or on the ceilings, walls, and floors of homes that have moisture management problems.

As mold and mildew grow, they produce a musty and unpleasant odor, especially in unaired places. These odors can permeate a room and become difficult to eliminate, even after addressing the mold problem. The presence of these odors can definitely make the living area less comfortable.

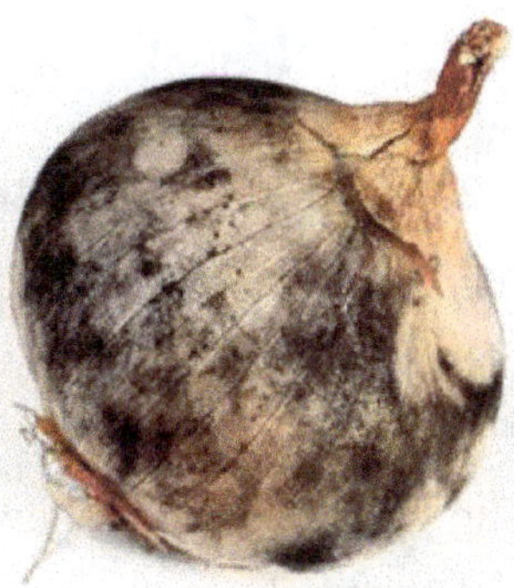

Some species of molds, like *Aspergillus versicolor* and *Stachybotrys chartarum*, commonly known as black mold, produce mycotoxins. This can result in health issues ranging from irritation of the mucous membranes, skin rashes, allergies, and nausea to more serious issues, including suppression of the immune system, acute or chronic liver damage, central nervous system damage, endocrine effects, and cancer.

To detect mold in your house, scrutinize moist and dark areas since this is where it most commonly occurs. Look behind the refrigerator, washer, dryer, and around the hot water heater. Check if there is any discoloration that could hint at the beginning of an upcoming infestation. Touch the walls to see if they feel moist. This would indicate a potential problem area. Sometimes, mold and mildew can contaminate the air conditioning system and heat ducts. Thus, they should be periodically inspected and cleaned. Take immediate action to remediate potential problems before they become a health issue.

To prevent mildew and mold problems, repair water leaks promptly, improve ventilation, and maintain proper humidity levels. The best preventative measure is to regularly inspect those areas where mildew and mold are most likely to grow. This will prevent damage to the house as well as reduce the possibility of health issues.

Bacteria And Viruses

The smallest organisms that inhabit our homes are bacteria and viruses. Although they cannot be seen with the naked eye, they can still have significant impacts on our health and well-being. Good hygienic practices, such as thoroughly washing your hands after you use the restroom and taking frequent showers, can help prevent contracting bacterial and viral infections.

The most common germ-infested object in the home is the kitchen cleaning pad. Most people do not rinse them well when they are done using them, giving the microbes plenty of nutrients to grow on. Areas in the home that are frequently contaminated are the bathrooms and kitchens because they contain many surfaces that are frequently touched. However, other objects, such as handheld electronics, smartphones, and even money, are high-touch items that can potentially be fomites that transmit pathogens to a host. Also, air conditioning and heating ducts may contain high numbers of microorganisms.

There are four genera of bacteria that are common in households: Staphylococcus, Micrococcus, Pseudomonas, and Bacillus. Staphylococcus aureus can result in skin infections, food poisoning, and nasal infections. Some strains, such as methylene-resistant Staphylococcus aureus (MRSA), are multiple-drug resistant. Micrococcus luteus can be found in meat products, water, and soil. It can cause septic arthritis, prosthetic valve endocarditis, and recurrent bacteremia in the circulatory system. Bacillus cereus can adhere to airborne dust particles, although it does not commonly cause respiratory infections. However, it is a common cause of food-borne gastroenteritis. Pseudomonas aeruginosa is highly contagious and can cause bacteremia that can result in infections of the ears, eyes, lungs, skin, and urinary tract. Immunocompromised individuals are especially susceptible to bacterial and viral diseases. It most frequently occurs in moist areas such as sinks or baths.

All species of bacteria should be considered to be potential opportunistic pathogens. This means that they may normally be harmless but can cause disease under the right environmental conditions. While bacteria can usually be easily treated by antibiotics and antiseptics, some strains of bacteria have developed resistance to them, and they are, therefore, difficult to treat. Thus, prevention is the best way to deal with microorganisms.

Beds can harbor bacteria if not properly cleaned. Studies have found that hospital beds routinely contain several potentially pathogenic species of Staphylococcus, including Staphylococcus aureus. Bed linens left unwashed for extended periods become breeding grounds for various types of microorganisms. One study found that pillowcases and sheets contained millions of bacteria per square inch after only four weeks of use without laundering.

Our skin is a host to both beneficial and potentially harmful microbes. On any given day, the average person's body is home to about 1 trillion bacteria across the skin's surface. While most coexist peacefully, some bacteria provide benefits, such as preventing the colonization of pathogens. However, opportunistic pathogens can enter the body through breaks in the skin and cause infections. Maintaining the appropriate hygienic practices, including frequent handwashing and cleaning heavily trafficked surfaces, will help control the spread of microbes within our homes and between individuals. It better enables our protective microbiomes to flourish while minimizing risks from disease-causing microorganisms. Once again, awareness is the key to minimizing health issues. Pathogenic bacteria have been found to persist for up to two weeks on inanimate objects such as clothing, sheets, and towels. This includes Escherichia coli and Staphylococcus aureus. Even more concerning, influenza viruses have been detected on fabrics for over 12 hours. Other viruses, such as Norovirus, which causes stomach flu, have been found to survive for up to 10 days.

Another consideration regarding pathogenic microorganisms is viruses that may be found in our homes. Fortunately, viruses are usually susceptible to environmental conditions and usually die off relatively quickly. Rhinovirus, which causes colds, can last up to one hour on human hands. Respiratory Syncytial Virus (RSV) can live for up to six hours on door handles. On hard surfaces, parainfluenza viruses can last for 10 hours, while influenza viruses can remain for up to 24 hours on hard surfaces. Coronaviruses such as COVID-19 can survive for several days, especially in cold, dry environments. In these time periods, people can be exposed when they come into contact with these contaminated surfaces. Another mode of transmission is via respiratory droplets, which can travel 18 feet when people cough or sneeze. The solution to minimizing exposure to indoor viruses is to frequently replace cleaning pads, disinfect hard surfaces where they may be found, keep the house clean, and aerate the house regularly. Practicing good hygiene will also help minimize viral exposure.

Luckily, most pathogens do not live for very long outside the human body. The environment is a harsh place, and they have yet to adapt survival strategies. Relatively few viruses or bacteria can cause a disease in a susceptible person. Thus, keeping the home clean, regularly washing reusable fabrics with hot water and dryer heat, disinfecting hard surfaces like countertops, and frequent and thorough handwashing will minimize the spread of harmful microorganisms.

CHAPTER 4: CHEMICAL HAZARDS IN YOUR LIVING SPACE

Various types of chemicals are used for cleaning purposes, and most people are not aware of their potential problems, how to safely use them, or how to properly store them to prevent harm to themselves and their family members. Some of these chemicals can be dangerous if not handled properly. Therefore, it is important to discuss the hazards associated with household chemicals and how best to manage them.

Asbestos, commonly found in older homes, is composed of silicon, a naturally occurring element. As a fibrous mineral, asbestos could be easily spun into threads and woven into mats or ropes. Its heat resistance and insulation properties made it highly prized. Asbestos was used in a variety of applications, including insulation for pipes and ducts, fireproof roofing, brake linings, and heat-resistant textiles. Its versatility led to widespread use in buildings constructed in the early and mid-1900s.

There are six types of asbestos. The three most commonly used were Chrysotile (White Asbestos), which accounts for 90% of the asbestos used in products like asbestos cement, gaskets, brakes, brake linings, other vehicle friction products, and roof shingles; Grunerite (Amosite or Brown Asbestos), utilized in fire-resistant materials; and Crocidolite (Blue Asbestos), commonly found in pipe insulation. The other three types—Anthophyllite, Tremolite, and Actinolite asbestos—were less commonly used.

Initially, the health risks associated with asbestos exposure were not well understood. Over time, asbestos becomes friable, meaning its fibers become brittle and easily crumble into microscopic particles that can become airborne. When inhaled, these fibers deeply penetrate the lungs, where they can remain because the respiratory system cannot expel them. Asbestos fibers do not break down, leading to scarring of lung tissue and causing diseases such as asbestosis and malignant mesothelioma, which can take decades to develop. Asbestos is classified as a Category 1 human carcinogen, responsible for more than 90,000 deaths globally each year, with many more people suffering from asbestosis.

The widespread use of asbestos has been a significant factor in the rise of lung cancer cases in the United States. Asbestos particles accumulate in the lungs, reducing their vital capacity. I have witnessed individuals with asbestosis who could not walk across a room without becoming breathless, as if they had just completed a marathon. After 30 to 40 years, lung cancer or mesothelioma may develop. The fibers are so small that they can migrate from the lungs to other parts of the body, where they accumulate and cause additional harm.

During my career as an environmental toxicologist, I investigated numerous sites where improper asbestos handling endangered lives. One notable case involved a former horse racing track, where asbestos waste from a nearby factory had been used as a sub-surface cushion for the racetrack. However, the horses' hooves disturbed the ground, releasing asbestos fibers into the air. Many trainers, stable hands, and other workers subsequently developed asbestos-related lung diseases from inhaling these fibers. It wasn't until 1989 that the Environmental Protection Agency (EPA) finally banned the use of asbestos.

The catastrophic collapse of the Twin Towers on 9/11 was a tragedy with far-reaching health consequences. In addition to the immediate loss of life, many rescue workers and first responders later developed serious health issues, including cancer, due to asbestos exposure during the rescue operations. The World Trade Center, constructed before the 1989 asbestos ban, contained large quantities of asbestos fireproofing materials. On that tragic day, the falling debris and dust clouds released high levels of asbestos throughout lower Manhattan. In the aftermath, many first responders and volunteers searched through the wreckage without proper respiratory protection. Tragically, twice as many 9/11 workers have died from toxic exposures as the 2,974 people who perished on that day.

Lead is commonly found in older residential and industrial buildings, where it was once used extensively in paint to increase durability and in plumbing pipes. It was also added to gasoline to boost octane levels, allowing engines to run more smoothly. However, lead is highly toxic, particularly to children and pregnant women.

In adults, lead exposure can lead to serious health issues such as anemia, hypertension, kidney damage, immunotoxicity, and reproductive toxicity. For children, the effects are even more severe, including slowed growth and development, cognitive impairments, learning and behavioral problems, and hearing and speech difficulties. The most common ways children are exposed to lead are by inhaling or ingesting lead-contaminated paint chips or dust. Prolonged lead exposure in adults has also been linked to cancer and chronic organ damage. Recognizing the dangers, the EPA banned lead-based paint in 1978.

Homes containing asbestos or lead-based paint must be remediated to protect the health of their occupants. While removing asbestos from older homes can be costly, leaving it in place poses significant risks. Investing in the removal of these hazards is crucial for the health and well-being of residents—human life is worth the financial sacrifice.

Household Cleaners

Cleaning is essential for maintaining a fresh and sanitary home, but it's equally important to handle cleaning products with care. Many household cleaners contain potent chemicals that can pose significant health risks if misused or mishandled. While most people store their cleaning supplies under the kitchen sink, it's easy to become complacent about the potential dangers of these seemingly harmless bottles and containers over time.

Reading product labels is crucial, no matter how familiar you are with the brand or how long you've used them. Pay close attention to warnings like "poison," "danger," or "flammable," which signal the need for extra precautions. Labels often specify protective measures, such as wearing gloves, ensuring proper ventilation, or avoiding direct contact with skin and eyes. Adhering to these instructions can greatly reduce the risk of exposure.

Common household cleaners include bleach, which can release toxic fumes and cause skin and eye irritation as well as respiratory problems. Ammonia can lead to respiratory issues and skin irritation, and it becomes highly toxic when mixed with bleach. Drain cleaners are corrosive and can cause burns, eye damage, and respiratory issues.

Pesticides, which are neurotoxins, carcinogens, and endocrine disruptors, pose serious risks to humans and pets, including cancer. Air fresheners contain Volatile Organic Compounds (VOCs) that can trigger headaches, asthma attacks, respiratory difficulties, dermatitis, and neurological issues in sensitive individuals. Other cleaning products, such as paint and paint thinners, are also VOCs linked to headaches, dizziness, bone, brain, and nerve damage, as well as kidney disease. Furniture polish can cause vomiting, low blood pressure, pain in the throat, mouth, eyes, and ears, agitation, confusion, and dizziness. Oven cleaners, which are corrosive, can cause severe burns, eye damage, and respiratory problems.

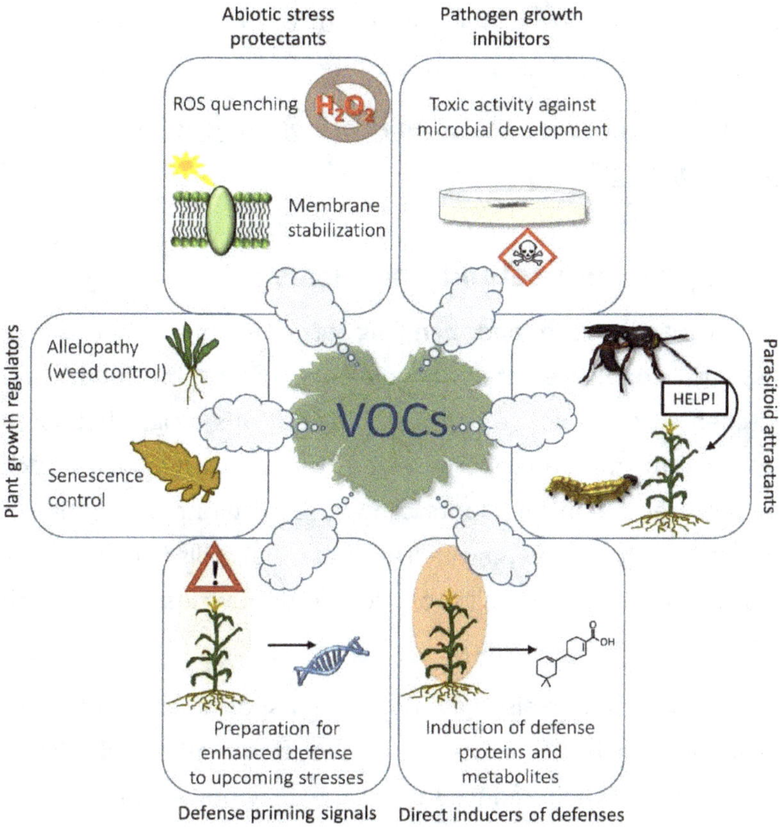

Oven cleaners are among the most hazardous products used in the home. The harsh fumes from the lye or acids they contain can quickly overwhelm a person in an enclosed space if proper safety measures are not taken. Reports of accidental poisonings and deaths from improper use underscore the importance of treating all household cleaning products, even familiar ones, as potential safety threats.

Using common sense is vital. Avoid placing your head in confined areas while spraying or saturating surfaces with strong cleaners. Following the manufacturer's safety instructions will minimize health risks. Being aware of the dangers inherent in these products will help keep you safe.

As the old adage goes, "***An ounce of prevention is worth a pound of cure.***"

Storage of Household Chemicals

Proper storage and handling of cleaning chemicals are essential for home safety. If you open the cabinet under the kitchen sink and notice odors wafting out, it's a sign that some bottles may not be properly sealed. This poses significant risks, as airborne chemical vapors can cause respiratory irritation if inhaled regularly and may indicate potential spills from unstable containers. Make sure all products are tightly closed after each use to prevent such issues.

Organization is also key. Dedicate a specific shelf solely for cleaning supplies, separate from other frequently used kitchen items. This will help reduce the risk of accidental exposure.

In case of an accident, emergency contact information is usually clearly displayed on the container. This information is crucial for responders who may need to identify the contents of a bottle quickly. The label will include the ingredients and manufacturer information, which can help facilitate appropriate medical care if problems arise from accidental exposure.

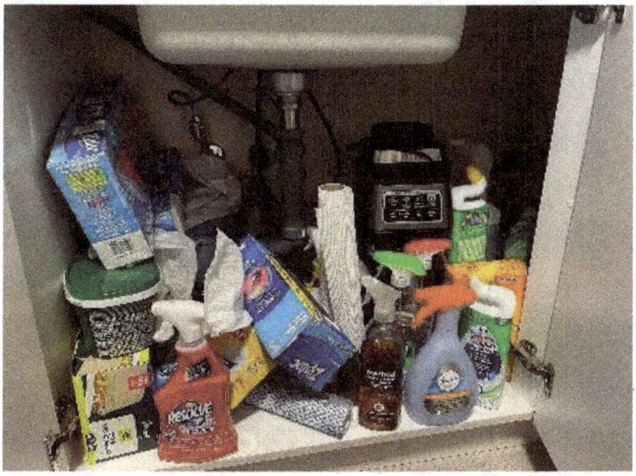

Expiration dates are another often-overlooked aspect of household chemical safety. Just as food and medicine degrade over time, household cleaners also have expiration dates. Discard any products that have expired; using unstable ingredients that may no longer work properly or may have become hazardous is not worth the risk. If you are unsure how to properly dispose of these products, contact your local health agency for guidance.

Even relatively minor exposures can result in temporary lung irritation or skin redness. With a bit of diligence, the dangers posed by household products can be minimized. Always observe proper precautions with each chemical task you undertake. If you are unsure of a product's potential risks, protect your skin and eyes and work in well-ventilated spaces. Numerous reports highlight tragedies caused by exposure to toxic fumes or mishandling of chemicals in confined areas, so take every precaution seriously.

Symptoms That May Indicate Exposure To Household Chemicals

It's essential to recognize the potential dangers of chemical exposure and understand how to handle such situations effectively. Chemical contact with the skin can cause irritation or absorption into the bloodstream, while volatile chemicals can be easily inhaled, leading to respiratory issues. Common signs of overexposure include dizziness, lightheadedness, coughing, shortness of breath, nausea, headaches, and irritation of the eyes, nose, or throat. Prolonged exposure to even low concentrations of toxic chemicals can result in a gradual decline in health, so vigilance is key.

Taking swift action can greatly improve outcomes. If toxic chemicals come into contact with the skin, immediately rinse the affected area thoroughly to remove the substance and prevent absorption. In cases of inhalation exposure, move the individual to a well-ventilated area to breathe fresh air, allowing Volatile Organic Compounds (VOCs) to dissipate quickly. For those experiencing nausea or dizziness, have them sit down with their head lowered between their knees to promote blood flow to the brain, and consider applying a cold, damp cloth to the forehead to alleviate discomfort. These steps can help stabilize the individual until proper medical care is available.

Always keep the Poison Control Hotline number readily accessible: 800-222-1222. Available 24/7, this resource can help prevent over 75% of unnecessary emergency room visits due to accidental poisoning and reduce the risk of severe outcomes. When consulting the hotline, provide accurate details, as their guidance is based on understanding the specific situation.

Recommendations may range from self-care at home to the immediate dispatch of an ambulance. No case is too minor or severe to warrant a call to the Poison Control Center.

By taking necessary precautions and staying aware, you can handle household products with greater confidence. Being proactive will help protect you and your loved ones should any issues arise in the home.

CHAPTER 5: INDOOR AIR POLLUTION

Indoor air pollution is particularly significant because most people spend about 90% of their time indoors, whether at home or in an office. This issue is exacerbated by the increasing use of synthetic building materials. Indoor air pollution arises from the presence of pollutants such as volatile organic compounds (VOCs), particulate matter, inorganic compounds, physical chemicals, and biological factors. High concentrations of these pollutants can significantly degrade indoor air quality and negatively impact human health.

Following the COVID-19 pandemic, people now spend more time at home than in the past. Additionally, electronic devices enable us to complete many tasks remotely while staying indoors. Although atmospheric pollution is addressed by various health agencies, indoor air quality often receives insufficient attention.

Indoor air pollution can affect health both in the short term and long term. Poor indoor air quality is linked to approximately 4.3 million deaths each year.

Indoor air quality (IAQ) refers to the quality of the air within and around buildings as it relates to the health and comfort of the occupants. The quality of the air we breathe indoors has become an increasingly important health and environmental concern. Several factors contribute to decreased indoor air quality, some of which are recognizable by their distinctive odors. Two out of three common indoor air quality problems involve the HVAC system (heating, ventilation, and air conditioning).

Prolonged issues with this system can lead to serious health problems. The types of indoor air pollutants and the health problems they cause are discussed below.

Gases

Volatile Organic Compounds (VOCs)

Volatile organic compounds (VOCs) are substances with high vapor pressure, which means they readily evaporate into the atmosphere. Many VOCs are synthetic and are used or produced during the manufacture of various products. These compounds are found in numerous materials used to build and maintain homes, where they can be released into the indoor air we breathe. The EPA has found that concentrations of several common organic pollutants are two to five times higher indoors than outdoors. Consequently, spending most of our time indoors increases our exposure to these elevated airborne pollutants.

Common sources of VOCs in the home include paints, paint strippers, solvents, wood preservatives, aerosol sprays, cleansers and disinfectants, moth repellents, air fresheners, stored fuels, automotive products, hobby supplies, dry-cleaned clothing, pesticides, building materials, furnishings, craft materials, glues and adhesives, and permanent markers. Health effects from VOC exposure can include irritation of the eyes, nose, and throat; headaches; allergic skin reactions; loss of coordination; dizziness; shortness of breath; fatigue; nausea; nosebleeds; and damage to the liver, kidneys, and central nervous system. Additionally, exposure to VOCs is associated with an increased risk of cancer.

Common VOCs:

- **Acetone:** Commonly used as a nail polish remover and in furniture polish. It acts as an irritant and is considered a probable carcinogen.
- **Butanal:** Produced by burning candles, barbecues, and gas stoves. It primarily acts as an irritant and is not highly toxic.
- **Methylene chloride (dichloromethane):** Found in paint removers, aerosol solvents, and flame-retardant chemicals. It can cause numbness and tingling in the limbs, nausea, drowsiness, and dizziness, and is also a potent carcinogen.
- **Formaldehyde:** The most common VOC in the home, present in products such as plastics, lacquers, and carpets. It is both an irritant and a carcinogen.
- **Carbon disulfide:** Found in chlorinated tap water; it can harm the eyes, skin, nervous system, liver, kidneys, and heart.

Not all volatile compounds lead to adverse health effects. The potential health impact of an organic chemical depends on several factors, including its chemical structure, ability to be absorbed into the circulatory system, toxicity, concentration in indoor air, duration of exposure, and individual susceptibility.

Some volatile organics have a distinctive odor, such as hydrogen sulfide, which smells like rotten eggs. However, many of these gases are odorless, colorless, and tasteless, making them difficult to detect without specialized equipment.

Carbon Monoxide (CO)

Carbon monoxide (CO) poses a significant risk because it is undetectable without monitoring equipment, making its effects insidious. It is produced when there is insufficient oxygen in a room to generate carbon dioxide. Indoor sources of carbon monoxide arise from combustion processes such as cooking and heating. Potential sources include unvented kerosene and gas space heaters, leaky chimneys and furnaces, backdrafting from various appliances, gas stoves, generators, and tobacco smoke.

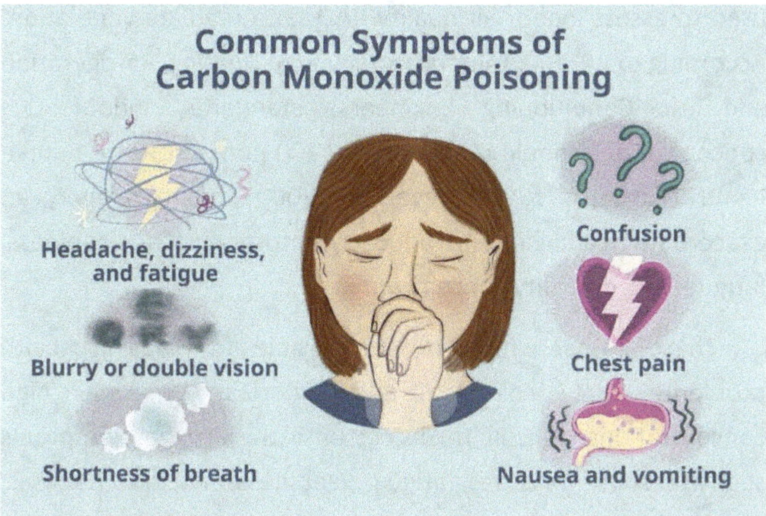

In areas without gas stoves, CO concentrations typically range from 0.5 to 5 ppm, while areas near gas stoves may exceed 30 ppm. The Permissible Exposure Limit (PEL) for CO is between 35 and 50 ppm. Exposure to CO can lead to adverse health effects, including fatigue, headaches, confusion, and dizziness, due to inadequate oxygen levels in the brain. At low concentrations, it can impact cardiovascular and neurobehavioral processes, while at high concentrations, it can cause unconsciousness or death.

Carbon Dioxide (CO_2)

Carbon dioxide (CO_2) is another colorless and odorless gas, constituting about 0.04% of the Earth's atmosphere. It is a human metabolite released during exhalation and is present in ambient air at an average concentration of approximately 400 ppm, primarily due to fossil fuel combustion. Indoor CO_2 levels are used to assess indoor air quality (IAQ) and regulate ventilation. According to ASHRAE (American Society of Heating, Refrigeration and Air Conditioning Engineers) standards, indoor CO_2 concentrations should remain below 700 ppm to ensure human health. Exposure to CO_2 levels of 3,000 ppm or higher can exacerbate headaches and induce symptoms such as sleepiness, fatigue, and difficulty concentrating.

These gases, which are responsible for causing health problems, are colorless and odorless, making high concentrations difficult to detect until they trigger symptoms such as respiratory issues, fatigue, sleepiness, and, in some cases, digestive problems.

Radon

Radon is a colorless and odorless radioactive gas produced from the natural radioactive decay of uranium found in rocks, soils, and water. It can also be present in building materials, water, and natural gas. Its impact on health, particularly its association with lung cancer, is significant. Radon exposure is estimated to contribute to between 3% and 14% of all lung cancer cases, with the risk increasing as radon concentrations rise. This indicates a linear dose-response relationship, showing a proportional increase in lung cancer risk with greater radon exposure.

Radon levels are typically higher indoors, especially in homes and workplaces. Factors such as local geology, building construction, and ventilation quality influence indoor radon levels. Radon enters buildings through cracks in floors and other openings, accumulating in basements, cellars, and ground-level living spaces.

To mitigate radon exposure, the World Health Organization (WHO) has implemented policies and regulations aimed at reducing its health risks. Effective methods for new and existing buildings include improved ventilation, sealing floors and walls, and installing radon sump systems. Passive mitigation systems can reduce indoor radon levels by over 50%, and further reductions can be achieved with the use of ventilation fans.

Particulate Contaminants

Dust

House dust is a heterogeneous mixture of substances and serves as a primary indicator of poor indoor air quality. It is composed of various particulate contaminants, which can be either solid or liquid and vary in size. The composition of house dust can differ from home to home but often includes textile fibers, grit and sand, insect fragments, pet dander, human and animal hair, food remnants, pollen, mold spores, bacteria, viruses, skin flakes, insulation material, and dust mites along with their excrement. Activities such as vacuuming, sweeping, cleaning carpets and upholstery, and disturbing curtains and blinds can stir up dust within the home.

Cooking, particularly frying, grilling, or baking, also contributes to airborne dust by releasing cooking oils, smoke, and food particles. Simply walking around the home can disturb settled dust, especially in areas with carpets and rugs. Each step can release dust particles trapped in floor coverings, increasing the overall dust load in the indoor environment. Homes with carpeting tend to have higher levels of house dust compared to homes without carpeting.

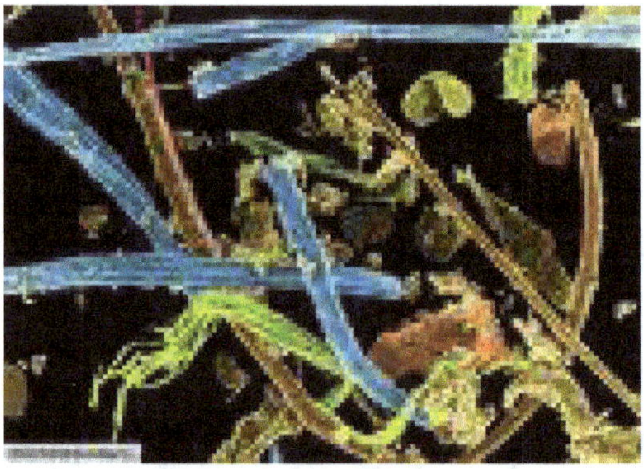

Additionally, dust can accumulate on draperies, decorative items, books, pets, upholstered furniture, and fireplaces. Inadequate cleaning methods, a lack of effective filtration systems, high foot traffic, geographical location, yard type, and the condition of central air systems all influence dust levels. Visible particles such as dirt, soot, or smoke can provoke irritation in the upper respiratory tract and exacerbate symptoms in individuals with allergies, asthma, or other respiratory conditions.

Dirt

Dirt particles can be found throughout the home and can easily enter indoor spaces through open windows and doors or be tracked in on shoes. These particles accumulate on surfaces such as furniture and objects, becoming airborne when disturbed, thus reducing indoor air quality.

Soot

Soot is a fine black powder composed of carbon particles resulting from incomplete combustion of organic matter like wood, coal, or oil. Indoor sources of soot include candles, cooking equipment, malfunctioning heating systems, and tobacco smoke. Soot particles can irritate the respiratory system and pose health risks, especially to those with existing respiratory conditions.

Smoke

Smoke is produced from incomplete combustion of fuel due to insufficient oxygen, leading to the creation of soot, tar, oils, ash, volatile organic compounds (VOCs), and fine particulates. Indoor sources of smoke include cooking, wood-burning stoves, fireplaces, and tobacco smoke. Prolonged exposure to indoor smoke can have serious health effects, including an increased risk of cancer, cardiovascular problems, and respiratory issues.

Respiratory Suspended Particulates (RSP)

Respirable and fine suspended particles include all solid and liquid particles in the air, many of which pose health risks. Particulate matter consists of a complex mixture of organic and inorganic particles varying in size, composition, and origin. Two major concerns for indoor air quality and health are PM2.5 and PM10:

- PM2.5: These are fine particles with a diameter of 2.5 µm or smaller. Due to their small size, PM2.5 particles can penetrate deeply into the lungs and potentially enter the bloodstream. Common indoor sources include combustion processes such as cooking, heating, and tobacco smoking. Outdoor pollutants can also infiltrate indoor spaces through ventilation systems, doors, and windows. Exposure to high levels of PM2.5 is associated with respiratory symptoms like coughing, wheezing, and shortness of breath and can exacerbate conditions such as asthma and chronic obstructive pulmonary disease (COPD). Long-term exposure is linked to cardiovascular diseases, lung cancer, and premature death.

- PM10: These are particles with a diameter of 10 µm or smaller. Although larger than PM2.5, PM10 particles can still pose health risks, particularly when inhaled in high concentrations. Indoor sources include dust from carpets, upholstery, and indoor construction activities. Outdoor sources such as vehicle emissions and industrial activities can also contribute to indoor PM10 levels. Inhalation of PM10 particles can irritate the respiratory tract, causing symptoms like coughing and throat irritation, and can worsen respiratory conditions. Long-term exposure may increase the risk of respiratory infections and cardiovascular diseases.

To mitigate health concerns related to airborne respiratory particles, proper ventilation is crucial for reducing particle concentrations and diluting indoor contaminants. Air purifiers with HEPA filters are effective in capturing particles like PM2.5 and PM10. Additionally, reducing indoor sources of particulate matter through regular vacuuming, dusting, and cleaning can help decrease particle levels. Maintaining control over airborne particulates, including PM2.5 and PM10, is essential for ensuring healthy indoor air quality and protecting respiratory health.

Indoor Allergens

The indoor environment contains numerous airborne allergens originating from both organic and inorganic sources. These allergens can exist as particles, vapors, or gases and primarily consist of large proteinaceous molecules. Some of the most prevalent indoor allergens include house dust, dust mites, animal dander, hair from cats and dogs, mice, cockroaches, and various types of fungi such as mildew and mold.

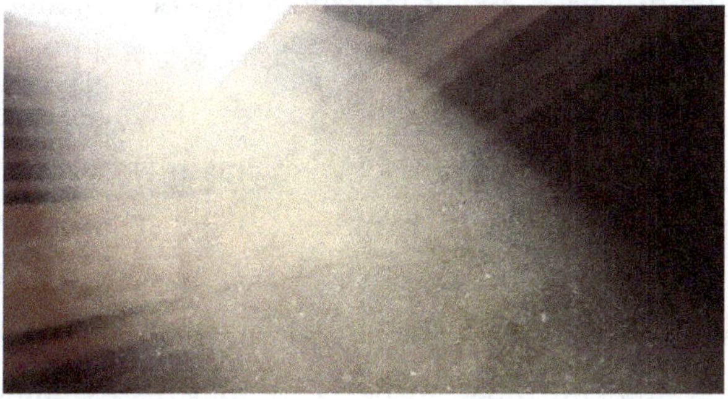

Dust Mites

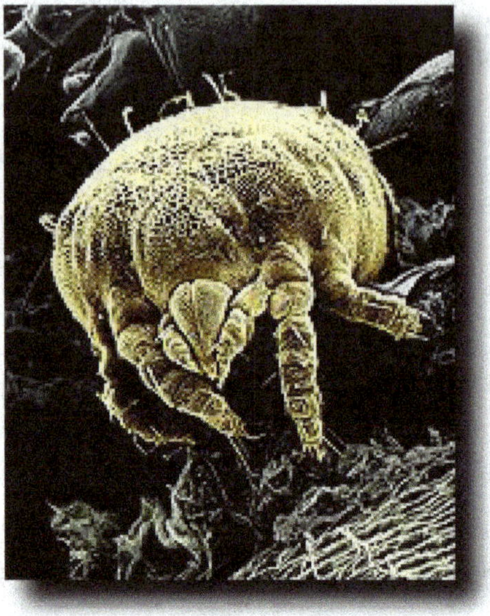

Dust mites are microscopically small creatures that resemble insects and thrive in dark, warm, and humid environments. They feed on living or dead human skin cells but do not bite, sting, or burrow into the body like some parasites. However, people can develop allergies to dust mites by inhaling their feces, urine, or decaying bodies. Allergic reactions to dust mites typically manifest as inflammation of the nasal passages, commonly known as a dust allergy. Dust mites are prevalent in almost every household and can thrive in bedding, mattresses, upholstered furniture, carpets, and even curtains.

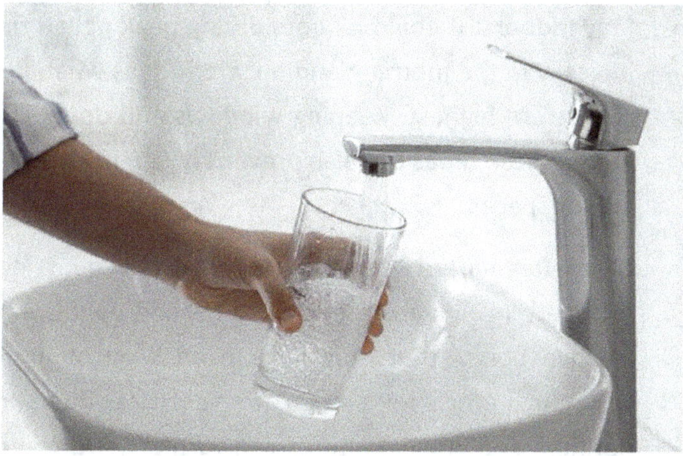

The level of humidity in a house plays a crucial role in determining the presence of high dust mite populations, as they rely on moisture from the air for survival. Unlike pet allergens, dust mite allergens typically do not remain airborne but rather settle quickly. Bedding is the most prevalent source of exposure because people spend hours asleep, inhaling these allergens.

Pollen

Pollen is a fine, granular substance found in the flowers of various trees, grasses, and weeds. It plays a crucial role in plant fertilization and can be dispersed by insects or carried by the wind. Many people develop allergic reactions to pollen, resulting in symptoms commonly associated with hay fever, such as a runny nose, itchy throat, and watery eyes. In severe cases, pollen exposure can lead to asthma.

While it is impossible to completely avoid pollen exposure, there are steps that can be taken to minimize allergic reactions:

- **Stay Indoors:** Remain indoors during peak pollen times, typically in the morning and on windy days when pollen counts are highest. Keeping windows and doors closed during these times can also prevent pollen from entering indoor spaces.
- **Clean Regularly:** Regularly clean and vacuum indoor surfaces, including carpets, curtains, and upholstery, to remove pollen that may have been brought indoors. Using high-efficiency particulate air (HEPA) filters in air purifiers and HVAC systems can further reduce indoor pollen levels.
- **Protect Yourself Outdoors:** When spending time outside, wear sunglasses and a wide-brimmed hat to protect your eyes and face from pollen. Shower and change clothes immediately upon returning indoors to remove any pollen particles that may have adhered to your body or clothing.
- **Monitor Pollen Forecasts:** Regularly check pollen forecasts and stay informed about pollen levels in your area to plan outdoor activities accordingly.

Pollen levels inside the home can vary depending on the season and location. Pollen can enter the home through vents, open windows, or by clinging to clothing. During peak pollen season, there can be a significant amount of pollen in the indoor air, although the concentration is typically lower compared to outdoor levels. Since most people spend a substantial portion of their day indoors, indoor pollen exposure should be considered.

Mold

Mold is a fungus that can grow on walls, ceilings, and floors, penetrating and deteriorating the materials it inhabits. It thrives in damp environments, often caused by leaks in roofs, windows, pipes, or flooding. These moist areas create ideal conditions for mold growth, which can lead to health problems such as respiratory infections, asthma, and severe allergies. Even if you are not allergic to mold, the presence of mold spores in the air can cause respiratory irritation or inflammation. Individuals with weakened immune systems are more susceptible to the effects of mold exposure, and it can exacerbate pre-existing health conditions. Mold is a natural part of our ecosystem and has been present for millions of years. It can enter homes through open doors, windows, and vents, and it may be found in heating and air conditioning systems. Mold can appear as spots and may have a noticeable odor.

If you suspect the presence of mold in your home, it is important to address the issue promptly. Professional mold remediation may be necessary to safely remove the mold and address the underlying moisture problem to prevent its recurrence. Additionally, maintaining proper ventilation and controlling indoor humidity levels can help prevent mold growth in the first place.

Mildew

Mildew refers to mold or fungus that typically grows on surfaces with high moisture levels. While the term "mildew" is often used to describe mold growth, mildew is specifically found on surfaces such as shower walls, windowsills, and other areas prone to dampness. Mildew is considered a surface fungus and can usually be cleaned and removed with household disinfectants. In contrast, mold growth often indicates a larger underlying issue and can be more invasive, potentially causing structural damage if not addressed properly.

Mildew typically appears as a patch of gray or white fungus on a moist surface and may sometimes have a powdery texture. It can also present as small, flat black spots.

Harmful Effects of Mold and Mildew

The presence of mold and mildew can pose significant risks to health and the surrounding environment. Some of the harmful effects associated with mold and mildew include:

Health Concerns: Mold and mildew can trigger various health issues, especially in individuals with specific sensitivities, allergies, or respiratory conditions. Symptoms may include coughing, wheezing, nasal congestion, throat irritation, and respiratory distress. Mold can also cause allergic reactions, leading to skin irritation, rashes, hives, nosebleeds, and migraines. Exposure to Aspergillus flavus and Aspergillus parasiticus can result in respiratory infections or exposure to their mycotoxins, which are strong carcinogens.

Structural Damage: Mold and mildew thrive in damp and humid conditions and can cause significant damage to wood, drywall, and insulation over time. This can result in costly repairs or demolition in severe cases.

Odor: Both mold and mildew emit a musty odor that can be difficult to eliminate. The presence of this odor often indicates an underlying mold issue. Eliminating the mold is the only way to prevent further growth and remove the associated odors.

Aesthetics: Visible mold growth is unsightly and detracts from the aesthetic appeal of a home. It can discolor surfaces, leave stains, and create an unappealing appearance.

To mitigate the risks associated with mold and mildew, it is crucial to address any moisture issues promptly. This includes identifying and fixing leaks, improving ventilation, and maintaining proper humidity levels in indoor spaces.

Controlling Mold and Mildew Growth

Mold and mildew can be controlled. The primary step to prevent mold from infiltrating your home is to maintain the humidity level as low as possible, ideally no higher than 50%. Recognizing signs of growth is crucial; visible indicators include warping and discoloration of household materials, along with a noticeable musty odor. Pay attention to changes in your environment and remain vigilant, especially in humid regions where mold can proliferate rapidly.

- **Proactive Measures:** Taking proactive steps to control mold growth is essential. Installing an air conditioner or dehumidifier can help maintain low humidity levels. A humidity meter from a home improvement store allows you to monitor levels regularly as they fluctuate throughout the day. Regularly inspecting plumbing fixtures, roofs, and foundations for leaks or water damage is vital to prevent moisture buildup, which is a catalyst for mold growth.

- **Proper Ventilation:** Proper ventilation in moisture-prone areas such as bathrooms, kitchens, and basements is critical for reducing humidity and promoting airflow. Installing exhaust fans in these areas and ensuring clothes dryers vent outside helps expel excess moisture. Promptly addressing water leaks or spills and thoroughly drying affected areas within 24-48 hours can prevent mold growth and minimize water damage.

- **Moisture Control:** In persistently moist areas like basements or crawl spaces, consider using waterproofing techniques and moisture-resistant materials. Regular cleaning and maintenance of HVAC systems, air ducts, and humidifiers can also prevent the spread of mold spores. By implementing these measures and remaining vigilant for signs of moisture intrusion, homeowners can effectively manage mold growth and maintain a healthy indoor environment for themselves and their families.

Pet Dander

Pet dander, often overlooked as an indoor pollutant, presents a significant problem for many allergy sufferers. It comprises tiny flecks of skin and hair shed by household pets. Even breeds advertised as hypoallergenic or low-shedding can produce dander, triggering allergy symptoms in sensitive individuals.

It's crucial to differentiate between animal dander and hair shedding. While hair shedding contributes to dander levels, dander primarily consists of skin cells. These microscopic particles can become suspended in indoor air, causing allergic reactions when inhaled or when they come into contact with sensitive individuals. Pet hair, though it can carry allergens like dander, is not as significant a source of allergens. Allergic reactions to pet dander vary from mild to severe and include symptoms such as coughing, sneezing, watery eyes, nasal congestion, and, in extreme cases, chest tightness or difficulty breathing. These symptoms can be sufficiently severe to impact the quality of life for allergy sufferers, necessitating measures to reduce exposure to pet dander at home. Poor indoor air quality can further exacerbate allergy symptoms. Factors like air temperature, humidity levels, and airflow influence allergen dispersion and, subsequently, the severity of allergic reactions.

Understanding the distinction between animal dander and hair shedding and taking steps to minimize exposure can alleviate allergy symptoms and enhance the comfort of individuals living with pets.

Insects

Indoor air pollution can have another unexpected contributor: insect pests. Similar to rodents, insects often carry allergens into your home. Not only can they harbor pathogenic bacteria and viruses, posing direct health risks, but their body parts can also act as allergens.

Cockroaches, in particular, are notorious for this, as their bodies, shells, droppings, and saliva can trigger severe allergies and asthma. Even dead roaches can trigger an allergic reaction. Other common indoor insect pests can also pose health risks. For instance, the fecal matter of dust mites contains proteins that can trigger allergic reactions and exacerbate asthma symptoms.

Household pests like ants, flies, and beetles can carry pathogens, potentially contaminating food and surfaces. Thus, insects should be excluded from our homes as much as possible. Several strategies can be implemented to improve indoor air quality and mitigate health risks associated with insect pests. Regular cleaning, especially in insect-prone areas, reduces food sources and breeding grounds. Sealing cracks and gaps in walls, floors, and windows prevent pest entry. Proper food storage and waste management deter infestations. In severe cases, professional pest control services may be necessary for effective elimination and prevention of recurrence.

Ways To Improve Indoor Air Quality (IAQ)

Let's start by assessing the air quality in our homes, a crucial step in ensuring the well-being of those who spend most of their time indoors. Determining whether the air quality at home and work is compromised is essential. You can take the initiative and conduct tests yourself if you're confident in your abilities, or alternatively, you can enlist the services of a professional to inspect your house.

Testing kits are available for purchase online, allowing you to check for various pollutants such as carbon monoxide, carbon dioxide, mold and mildew, radon, pollen, airborne particulates, and dust mites. However, if you seek a comprehensive assessment of your home, including volatile organic compounds, consulting an expert is advisable. While professional inspections incur charges, they provide in-depth insights into pollutant sources and offer advice on elimination or control measures. By conducting air quality tests, either independently or with professional assistance, you gain valuable information to safeguard your indoor environment and promote a healthier living space for yourself and your loved ones.

Keep Your House Clean

The most critical strategy to minimize airborne pollution is regular house cleaning. Dust accumulation is continuous, so maintaining a dust-free environment is essential for a healthy home. A healthy house should not have a visible layer of dust in corners.

For homes with carpeting, frequent vacuuming of carpets and rugs is necessary. Opting for hard surface floors instead of carpeting can reduce allergens. Regular decluttering is also important, as clutter traps dust and harbors insects.

While certain indoor plants like Ficus, Peace Lily, and Rubber plants are touted for their air-purifying qualities, they can also promote mold growth and harbor dust. If indoor allergens are a concern, it's advisable to avoid these plants.

Indoor plants can exacerbate allergies by releasing allergenic pollen and harboring dust and mold. Some plants contain latex in their sap, which can cause skin irritation upon contact and respiratory symptoms if inhaled. Common culprits include grasses, weeds, and trees that release pollen indoors, as well as plants with fine hairs or sap that provoke allergic reactions.

Careful selection of indoor plants is crucial for allergy sufferers, especially those allergic to pollen, dust, and mold. Choosing non-allergenic plants can help maintain a healthier and more comfortable indoor environment.

Change Your Filters

If you have a forced-air heating system installed in your home, it's crucial to ensure that the filters are cleaned and changed every three months. While electrostatic filters can effectively trap dust and other airborne irritants, regular filter changes further reduce the amount of particulates, mold, bacteria, and viruses that you will inhale. Regular maintenance of your heating system's filters not only improves indoor air quality but also helps to maintain the system's efficiency and longevity.

Invest In An Air Purifier

According to experts, if you're allergic to indoor allergens and unable to address the root cause, utilizing a HEPA air purifier could be beneficial. Placing these devices in frequently used areas of the house can significantly reduce exposure to airborne pollutants, thus lowering the risk of future health problems and potentially reducing allergic responses to airborne pollutants.

While completely eliminating these airborne pollutants may not be feasible, reducing their presence can significantly improve your overall quality of life. Additionally, consider using a dehumidifier in areas prone to dampness, such as basements, to discourage the growth of mold and mildew. Proper ventilation in bathrooms is essential, and regularly cleaning any visible mold buildup on shower surfaces, fixtures, or walls is recommended to maintain a healthy indoor environment.

Improve Ventilation

Don't overlook the importance of inviting fresh air indoors, even during colder months. Periodically opening windows allows for the introduction of fresh air into the house and provides an opportunity for built-up gases to escape. Additionally, using ventilation hoods over the stove when cooking helps expel cooking fumes and other potential air contaminants, contributing to a healthier indoor environment.

Reduce Dampness

To mitigate health risks associated with indoor dampness, including mold growth and volatile organic compound emissions, it's crucial to address and reduce damp conditions in indoor spaces. Various factors contribute to indoor dampness, such as humid climates, leaky pipes or roofs, areas prone to water accumulation, and inadequate ventilation in steam-rich environments like bathrooms and kitchens. These conditions can exacerbate respiratory symptoms like coughing, wheezing, and asthma attacks.

To combat dampness, consider employing strategies like using a dehumidifier, activating fans or opening windows after showering or cooking, and identifying and remedying areas of water accumulation or moisture within your home. Indoor air quality in your living environment can be influenced by many factors, leading to both immediate and long-term health consequences. Conducting tests to assess indoor air quality can provide reassurance and insight into potential pollutants. Subsequently, implementing measures to prevent and mitigate pollutants will enhance indoor air quality and reduce associated health risks, promoting a healthier living environment overall.

Shoes Worn Indoors

Most people do not give much thought to wearing shoes indoors; however, perhaps they should. Shoes that are worn indoors can pick up various contaminants, which can then be carried into the home. Simply walking on the pavement can expose you to a variety of contaminants. This can include disgusting things like spit, animal feces and urine, and gum. There are many reasons to remove shoes when entering a home.

These include cultural and environmental considerations as well as problems from a cleanliness and health perspective, including:

Cultural Norms: In many cultures, it is customary to remove shoes before entering a home as a sign of respect and cleanliness. This includes Japan, India, Afghanistan, Pakistan, Iran, Turkey, Malaysia, Thailand, Myanmar, New Zealand, Italy, and many other countries as well. Interestingly, it appears that the more ancient the civilization, the more common it is to customarily remove your shoes when entering a home.

Comfort: Wearing shoes indoors is probably less comfortable than going barefoot or wearing indoor slippers or socks. However, it may be more comfortable to wear shoes if a person has foot issues or if the floor is cold. Indoor slippers may be helpful for people with foot problems because they can provide arch support, cushion your feet, and keep you warmer in the winter. Also, kicking them off when you get home can be an emotional stress reliever.

Also, shoes can cause foot problems such as 1) Influencing the structure of your feet, 2) Altering the position of your feet, and 3) Altering the mechanics of your feet. Conversely, many reflexologists feel that walking barefoot at home can improve blood circulation in your feet, help you sleep better, and even reduce pain and inflammation.

Cleanliness: Chemicals, toxic dust, germs, dirt, mud, and other debris can be tracked into the house from outdoor surfaces, which can soil carpets, rugs, and floors. Further, carpeting is able to retain a great deal of dust. This can lead to increased cleaning efforts as well as wear and tear on flooring materials. It is especially important to avoid wearing shoes in the house if you have young children. They could ingest germs or chemicals since they spend so much time on the floor. Thus, removing shoes indoors can help reduce these potential problems and maintain better hygiene.

Noise: Our home is supposed to be our sanctuary. A place where we are not disturbed. However, shoes, especially those with hard soles or high heels, can produce enough noise to disturb others, particularly in multi-story dwellings. As a courtesy to others, we should tread lightly or take off our shoes when we enter our home.

Flooring: Do not underestimate the toll your shoes can take on your floors. Hard-soled shoes, especially, can scratch, scruff, and even gouge hardwood, laminate, and tile floors. Sneaker soles can also scuff the flooring. This can result in aesthetic damage that may eventually require costly repairs or replacements.

Microorganisms: Shoes serve as a fomite, moving germs from one place to another. They can pick up microbes from various surfaces, including public restrooms, streets, and sidewalks, which can then be transferred to indoor surfaces, potentially leading to illnesses. This is especially true in households with vulnerable individuals, such as children or the elderly.

Clostridium difficile was found on at least 26% of the shoes that were tested, which can cause severe diarrhea and colon inflammation on the soles of their shoes. It is resistant to most household cleaners because it is a spore-former. Another pathogen found on shoes is Staphylococcus aureus, which can cause skin infections, meningitis, endocarditis, and more. The soles of your shoes can also carry Escherichia coli. Some strains of this bacterium, such as E. coli O157:H7, are virulent pathogens that can cause intestinal and urinary tract infections. You might be tracking into the house Staphylococcus aureus, which can cause boils, acne, and gastroenteritis. Other bacteria that have been isolated from shoes include Paracoccus, Rubellimicrobium, Janthinobacterium, Hymenobacter, and Rhodobacter. Some of these bacteria may be drug-resistant, making them even more dangerous.

It's even more important to take your shoes off indoors if you have carpet because it can hold more dust and bacteria than solid floors due to its greater surface area.

Microorganisms may live longer on the bottom of your outdoor shoes because shoes also pick up organic matter, which can serve as nutrients for bacteria to grow. Approximately 99% of the shoes that were tested were found to contain fecal material. Thus, your shoes are crawling with germs.

Chemicals: The ground is covered with residual toxins. Outdoor surfaces may contain pesticides, fertilizers, road salt, and particulates from automobile exhausts. These substances can be tracked indoors via your shoes. This can pose a health risk for the home's occupants, especially young children and pets. The toxicity of a poison depends on many factors. These include how much of the toxin you are exposed to, how long you have been exposed to it, how toxic it is, your overall health, and your lifestyle.

You're probably stepping on fertilizer, weed killer, and pesticides when you walk in fields, parks, gardens, and golf courses. Pesticide exposure can result in nose and throat irritation, dizziness, nausea, asthma, reproductive problems, and cancer. The World Health Organization estimates that about 385 million cases of pesticide poisoning occur annually worldwide, with at least 11,000 deaths. They are endocrine disruptors that can affect normal hormonal levels in your body.

Asphalt is another potentially toxic substance of concern. Newly laid asphalt has been shown to cause eye and respiratory irritation, lung and bladder cancer, heart disease, and reduced lung function. Fresh asphalt gives off airborne contaminants, including particulate matter, oil mist, and polycyclic aromatic hydrocarbons. Further, automobiles produce toxins such as gasoline, antifreeze, and toxic exhaust particulates. Your shoes can track traces of lead in the home if you live in an area with lead-contaminated soil or if you live in a home built before 1978 because of the presence of lead-based paint. In children, lead can cause mental retardation, hyperactivity, and stunted growth. Also, other toxic heavy metals like copper and zinc reside in the soils of urban parks and streets from decades of pollutants.

Per- and polyfluoroalkyl substances (PFAS) have been found to be carried on shoes. These are particularly concerning because they do not degrade. Unless you clean your house, they will remain on the floors. They have been associated with increased cholesterol levels, liver enzyme changes, lower infant birth weights, kidney or testicular cancer, decreased vaccine responses in children, and an increased risk of high blood pressure in pregnant women.

Allergens: Pollen, spores, and other allergens can cling to shoes and be brought indoors, exacerbating the allergy symptoms of sensitive individuals. Removing shoes upon entry could help to minimize the symptoms. In fact, you should wipe your shoes on a doormat before entering and then take them off once you are inside.

In conclusion, a no-shoes policy indoors can help to maintain cleanliness, reduce the spread of germs and allergens, prolong the lifespan of flooring, and promote a more comfortable and hygienic indoor environment. It can also be more comfortable when you remove your shoes. However, wearing shoes indoors is a personal choice that is made based on knowledge. You should consider wearing indoor slippers instead of shoes. There can be a designated area near the entrance where shoes can be removed and stored, and slippers can be obtained.

CHAPTER 6: THE WATER WE DRINK - SAFETY CONCERNS

Water is a vital resource for our survival, yet accessing clean water presents increasingly critical challenges. In many areas, water is not easily accessible, and even where it is plentiful, the quality of the water supply may be marginal. Despite its fundamental importance, water availability and quality are taken for granted.

Municipal Drinking Water

Municipal water, commonly called tap water, is supplied to homes and industries through underground pipes in most locations. However, older pipes were joined using lead solder. Over time, the lead in the solder leaches into the water, causing health risks. Despite purification and filtration processes, many toxic chemicals, including lead, remain in the drinking water supply.

Quality of Municipal Drinking Waters

Most municipal waters in the U.S. should not be assumed to be safe for consumption due to industrial and environmental pollution. It is widely acknowledged that all water sources contain some form of contamination. Consider the following facts:

- There are approximately 35,000 pesticides containing 600 chemical compounds, yet municipal water systems are only required to test for six of them. Many of these chemicals are known to cause birth defects, nerve damage, sterility, and cancer.

- The General Accounting Office reports that 20% of the nation's 65,000 community water systems fail to meet the minimum water quality standards set by the Safe Drinking Water Act.
- More than 700 organic chemicals have been identified in drinking water, and many of them are known or suspected carcinogens.

Degradation Of The Water Supply

Some river waters are sequentially utilized by multiple cities. For instance, the Huron River in Michigan flows over 125 miles from its headwaters at Big Lake, near Pontiac, to its mouth in Lake Erie. It serves as the drinking water supply for approximately 12 cities and townships. Each municipality withdraws water from the river, utilizes it, treats its wastewater, and then releases it back into the river. Subsequently, the next town downstream utilizes this water. Unfortunately, the quality of the water progressively deteriorates as it traverses from one city to the next. By the time it reaches Lake Erie, the water exhibits a strong odor and an unpleasant taste. Furthermore, it is contaminated with hexavalent Chromium, a potent carcinogen. Despite these issues, the EPA permits downstream residents to consume this water.

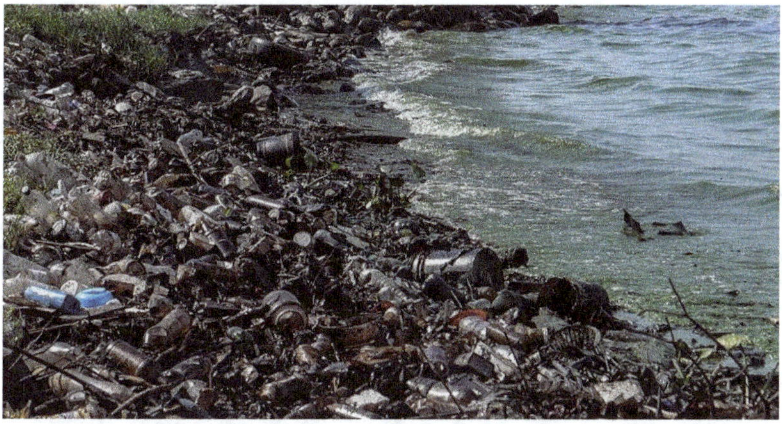

Contrary to expectations, if municipal water fails to meet the EPA's water quality standards, the water supply will not be terminated until the issues are rectified. Substandard water is still distributed to homes and industries because water is essential in cases where pathogens are detected in the water supply, and a directive to boil the water before consumption is issued. Additionally, the local water department is required to notify the public of any water quality issues. However, these notifications are often buried within lengthy informational reports about municipal drinking water. Consequently, few people are aware of the severity of the problem. Understanding the source and treatment of your water can provide insight into the quality of the water flowing from your faucet.

Degradation Of Water Quality

Human health can be jeopardized when the public assumes that the consumption of tap water is safe. Consider these Municipal Water Catastrophes:

- Flint, Michigan: The Flint water disaster, which began in 2014, gained nationwide attention due to elevated concentrations of lead detected in the city's water supply. This resulted from a change in water sources and inadequate corrosion management measures, leading to hundreds of residents being exposed to lead poisoning.
- Walkerton, Ontario: In May 2000, the town experienced an *Escherichia coli* outbreak in its municipal water, causing over 2,000 people to fall ill and resulting in seven deaths. The infection was related to agricultural runoff and was exacerbated by inadequate monitoring.
- Camp Lejeune, North Carolina: Soldiers and employees at the Camp Lejeune Army Base were exposed to carcinogenic levels of Trichloroethylene (TCE) and Perchloroethylene (PCE) in their drinking water due to leaking tanks and inappropriate waste disposal methods.

In households, tap water is used for various purposes, including washing dishes, cooking, showering, and watering lawns and plants. Surprisingly, less than one percent goes straight into our drinking glass. Hence, it is crucial to never overlook the quality of tap water. Therefore, understanding the potential problems associated with tap water is essential.

Drinking water undergoes treatment and processing to ensure that it meets the standards set by the Environmental Protection Agency (EPA). The EPA evaluates approximately 90 different parameters, including factors such as pH, water temperature, dissolved oxygen, turbidity, total suspended solids, organic carbon, and chlorophyll A. Tests are also conducted for fecal coliforms, which indicate sewage pollution, as well as other bacteria. The EPA maintains a Priority Pollutant List (PPL) containing 129 different toxins. However, it's important to note that many potentially harmful chemicals have not been tested. Consequently, the quality of drinking water may still be questionable, yet the public relies on the EPA to protect us against unwanted exposures.

Tap water typically comes from rivers, wells, and lakes, which serve as drinking water reservoirs. The quality of drinking water is dependent on factors such as the initial water quality and the age of the water treatment plant. While some areas effectively remove 99 percent of the listed contaminants, high initial levels may result in unacceptable pollutant levels.

However, many cities are only able to do the bare minimum that is required, which can affect their safety. Thus, there is a chance that the public water supply may contain contaminants that can affect your health. Also, some municipalities still use lead pipes to carry their water. Knowing where your water comes from and how it is treated can give you an idea as to the safety of your water.

If the municipal water is found to contain undue levels of toxins or unacceptable bacterial levels, the supply is not cut off. It is allowed to flow to all of the homes and industries in the city while the problem is remediated. The affected water authority is required by the EPA to issue a warning to the public that there is a problem with the water supply. However, these notifications are often buried within lengthy informational reports about municipal drinking water. Consequently, few people are aware of the severity of the problem. If there is a fecal bacterial overload, the public will be notified to boil the water before it is used. However, the contaminated water is still being used for showers, cooking, and washing dishes. The end result is that you can never be sure that the water flowing to your home is indeed safe to consume.

Therefore, it is prudent to use a whole-house water purification system to ensure that your water is safe. Using an under-the-sink water purification system is fine for the kitchen or bathroom but does nothing for showers and other activities where water is used. The two most common ways to treat household water are by reverse osmosis or by using a multi-stage water treatment system. Reverse osmosis will yield extremely high-quality water, but it is very expensive to purchase and maintain. The water quality does not have to be at this level. Therefore, the use of a multi-stage water treatment system is recommended. It consists of a pre-filter to remove sand, debris, and some bacteria; an activated carbon filter to remove organic compounds, and an ion exchange filter to remove inorganic compounds and heavy metals.

Municipal Water System Challenges

Municipal water systems rely on a complex network of canals, reservoirs, pipes, and other infrastructure. About 85% of these systems are owned by public utilities, while the remaining 15% are owned by smaller private entities.

Managing these water systems has its challenges. They face a myriad of obstacles related to water quality and system effectiveness, such as an aging infrastructure, pollution, and changing environmental conditions. These challenges require innovative solutions. Technological advancements and system design changes are helping water utilities overcome these challenges.

Understanding the key challenges is the first step in finding effective solutions to safeguard community water supplies for the future. By addressing these issues head-on, we can ensure the continued availability of clean and safe water for generations to come.

You can determine the quality of your local municipal water supply and the contaminants found in the water by going to www.ewg.org/tapwater/ and then scrolling down to enter your zip code or using Find Your State.

Inadequate Water Quality Standards

Municipal water isn't ideal for drinking. Although the public water supply undergoes purification and filtration processes and must meet the water quality standards set by the EPA, many toxic chemicals may be present.

The EPA only checks for some of the toxic substances that are on their Priority Pollutant List (PPL), which contains 129 toxic chemicals. However, most of the toxicants on this list are not tested for in drinking water supplies. Consequently, the quality of our drinking water remains questionable, yet the public relies on the EPA Drinking Water Standards to protect against undesirable exposures.

Degradation Of The Water Supply

Some river waters are sequentially utilized by multiple cities. For instance, the Huron River in Michigan flows over 125 miles from its headwaters at Big Lake, near Pontiac, to its mouth in Lake Erie. It serves as the drinking water supply for approximately 12 cities and townships. Each municipality withdraws water from the river, utilizes it, treats its wastewater, and then releases it back into the river. Subsequently, the next town downstream utilizes this water. As the river traverses from one city to the next, the quality of the water progressively deteriorates. By the time the Huron River reaches Lake Erie, it exhibits a strong odor and an unpleasant taste. Not only has the quality of the water substantially deteriorated, but it is also contaminated with Hexavalent Chromium, a potent carcinogen. Despite these issues, the EPA permits downstream residents to consume this water.

Deteriorating Water System Infrastructure

Challenges faced by municipal water systems often stem from an aging infrastructure, many of which was constructed at least 40 years ago. Unfortunately, most water utilities struggle with limited funding, which hampers their ability to maintain and upgrade their systems adequately. As infrastructure ages and maintenance falls behind, these systems become more prone to breakdowns and failures. Without regular upkeep, issues like flooding, water contamination, and other serious problems can arise, potentially causing significant damage and reducing the availability of clean water for the community.

Older pipes were typically soldered together using leaded solder. Over time, the lead can leach into the water being carried by the pipes. Additionally, seemingly minor issues like pipe leaks can have significant consequences. In fact, the US loses up to 6 billion gallons of treated water each day due to leaking pipes and water main breaks.

To address these challenges, communities are modernizing their water systems and replacing aging components. Advancements in water management, including the use of advanced controls and artificial intelligence, are helping communities manage their systems more effectively. Novel approaches are being explored to improve water quality and system efficiency. By embracing these modernization efforts, communities can better ensure the reliability and sustainability of their water supplies.

The Continuous Accessibility Of Water

Ensuring a continuous supply of water has become a crucial issue for many cities, especially in metropolitan areas where the population is growing because this causes consumption rates to rise. Many cities rely on groundwater as part of their water source. However, the groundwater aquifer is being depleted faster than it can be recharged.

Communities that are located near the ocean and are experiencing aquifer depletion may experience saltwater intrusion. The aquifer becomes brackish because the porous rock in the aquifer acts like a siphon, drawing in saltwater from the nearby ocean.

In states like California, water districts often need to obtain water from other areas to meet the state's growing demand. To address these challenges, communities are taking proactive measures such as exploring alternative water sources, implementing sustainable water practices, and revising their water supply plans to safeguard existing resources. By adopting these strategies, communities can ensure a more resilient and sustainable water supply for the future.

Groundwater Management

Around 30% of the world's freshwater comes from underground aquifers. In drier regions, this figure can rise to as much as 40% of the total water supply. Aquifers are essentially large underground stores of water found within permeable rock or sediment layers.

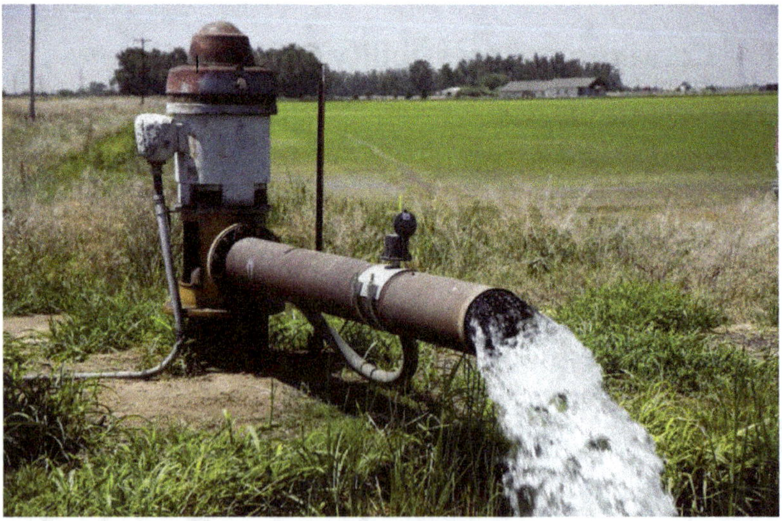

In heavily developed areas, extensive concrete surfaces prevent rainwater from seeping into the ground to replenish these aquifers. This increases the likelihood that an aquifer can become depleted. Additionally, some communities extract more water from their aquifers than can be naturally replenished through rainfall, leading to overuse and contamination. When groundwater is pumped out faster than it can be replenished, it can result in dry wells and pose significant challenges. This overuse can result in both aquifer depletion and a degradation of the quality of the groundwater. Water from industrial lagoons and contaminated surface runoff can find its way into the aquifers. This is particularly problematic during periods of drought.

Depleted aquifers can necessitate deeper well drilling, increasing the cost of the water supply. Aquifer depletion can result in saltwater intrusion because the porous rock that holds the groundwater acts as a siphon, drawing in saltwater from nearby oceans and resulting in increasingly brackish groundwater. Superficial aquifer depletion can also cause land subsidence, leading to the formation of sinkholes or sunken areas. Thus, it is important to manage groundwater resources to prevent these detrimental consequences from occurring.

Regulatory Compliance

Regulatory compliance regarding water quality and resource preservation is enforced by the United States Environmental Protection Agency (EPA), the Department of Health (DOH), and the Food and Drug Administration (FDA). However, despite increasing regulations aimed at safeguarding water, many cities face challenges keeping up due to limited staff, training, and funding. The bottled water regulations set forth by the FDA are less stringent than those set forth for municipal water by the EPA. This means that bottled water is not as closely regulated as tap water. Considering the fact that the EPA regulations are not very stringent, this is disconcerting and of great concern. Bottled water is regulated by the FDA (Food and Drug Administration) because it is considered a good sold in grocery stores. The FDA imposes fewer regulations on the safety of water consumption compared to municipal water. Companies have the freedom to bottle water as they see fit, with some even filling bottles with tap water.

States can set their own regulations, provided they are stricter than federal regulations. However, one in five states has not attempted to regulate bottled water. The lack of regulation is evident, as there is no standardized label required on bottled water for consumer safety due to the lack of regulation. Thus far, no studies have been done to determine if bottled water can affect human health.

These challenges can result in various issues within community water systems, including non-compliance with the Safe Drinking Water Act and other regulatory violations. To address these challenges, proactive management of contaminants and regular testing of water quality are essential. These measures provide opportunities to detect and manage contaminants effectively and identify and resolve potential problems before they escalate.

Lack of Financial Resources

As previously stated, many communities face the challenge of limited funds when it comes to improving their water management systems. Keeping water rates low is a priority. Customer attitudes also play a role. While people might not hesitate to pay for non-essential services like cable, they are frequently resistant to paying more for water because they view water as a right to which they are entitled. This creates a dilemma for water providers trying to balance the need for revenue with affordability for residents.

Finding additional funding is difficult since Federal and State grants and other resources are insufficient to satisfy the demand. Some communities have found success by forming strategic partnerships with other cities or by exploring unconventional funding options. By creating new paradigms, many municipalities have been able to tap into new financial resources and secure the capital needed to improve their water systems.

Bottled water, which is considered to be safe and environmentally friendly, has gained enormous popularity. However, bottled water poses intrinsic threats to human health.

The question is: Is bottled or municipal better to consume?

Bottled Versus Tap Water

Over the past few years, the consumption of bottled water has grown significantly. Bottled water is considered to be safe and convenient, and it is preferred over tap water. As a result, hydration has become a big business, with a surge in the number of bottled water production companies. There is now a wide array of choices available, including flavored water, alkaline water, carbonated water, distilled water, filtered water, artesian water, and spring water.

Bottled water is convenient, making it the top choice for many people. However, every convenience comes with a price. Bottled water production consumes a significant amount of energy used for the production of bottles, water treatment, bottling, transportation, and refrigeration. As a result, it is much more expensive than tap water. One gallon of tap water costs around a penny per gallon in the U.S., while a gallon of bottled water costs about $1.23.

Approximately 97.3% of all commercial water bottles are made of plastic due to its low manufacturing cost. About 600 billion plastic bottles and containers were produced globally in 2021, resulting in approximately 25 million tons of plastic waste. In the United States, about 50 billion water bottles are used annually, which requires 17 million barrels of oil for the production of the bottles. Also, this released at least 2 million tons of carbon dioxide into the atmosphere, contributing significantly to global warming.

Many toxins have been found to leach into bottled water due to the plastic that is used. Also, single-use water bottles that are discarded do not degrade. Thus, they remain in the environment for up to 400 years. During this time, they can break down into microplastics. To address this issue, municipalities have banned the sale of single-use plastic bottles, and some companies have begun using biodegradable bottles to reduce the environmental impact.

In the environment, plastic wastes break down into microscopic particles due to the action of solar radiation and ocean waves. Primary consumers can ingest these microplastics, which are then consumed by secondary consumers. This process leads to the spread and concentration of microplastics throughout marine life, ultimately returning to humans through fishing, consumption of fish, and contaminated water. It is estimated that marine animals ingest approximately 236,000 tons of microplastics a year. Over 100,000 marine animals have died due to the ingestion of microplastics. Recently, in Davao City, Philippines, a Cuvier-beaked whale that died was found to contain 88 pounds of plastic in its stomach. Preliminary studies indicated that 90% of seabirds have ingested plastic.

Chemical contaminants such as DEHA, a possible human carcinogen, and benzyl butyl phthalate (BBP), a potential hormone disruptor, can leach out of the bottles into the water they contain over time. The rate of leaching of these toxic chemicals depends on the temperature at which the bottles are stored and how long the water has been stored in the bottles. The higher the temperature and the longer the time of storage, the greater the concentration of toxic chemicals that will leach from the bottle into its contents.

Some of the toxic chemicals that may leach out of bottles into their contents are heavy metals, which can cause gastrointestinal problems, kidney dysfunction, nervous system disorders, birth defects, and cancer; Perfluoroalkyl and Polyflluoroalkyl Substances (PFAS), which can cause increased cholesterol levels, hormone disruption, a decrease in female fertility and an increase in hypertension during pregnancy; PET (Polyethylene terephthalate) can cause breast cancer, kidney damage, infertility, and other hormonal imbalances that can result in weight gain; BPA (Bisphenols) which can interfere with testosterone levels and is a hormone disruptor, possible cancer; and Phthalates which are potent carcinogens that can also disrupt testosterone and other hormone levels.

Despite the environmental concerns, water bottles offer undeniable convenience because they are lightweight, affordable, durable, and perfect for storage. However, single-use bottles are not the answer. Either bottles should be made of glass, which is inert, bottles should be produced that can be reused, or single-use water bottles should be made of biodegradable materials to prevent potential harm to human health and the environment.

Well Water

Many people believe that well water is healthy and does not pose any health risks because it comes from deep underground. However, this is not always true. For example:

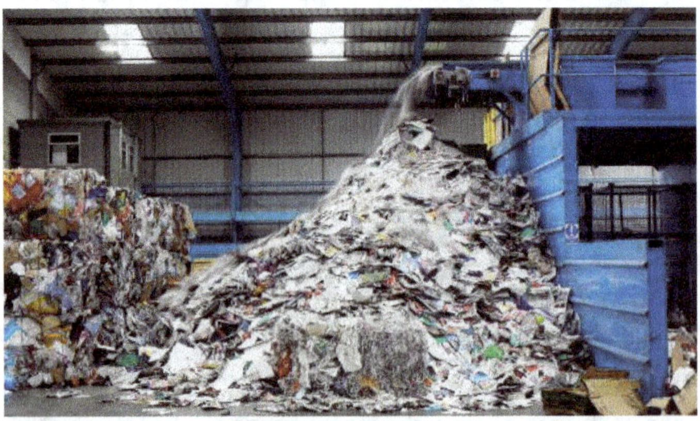

- **Franklin Borough, New Jersey** - Metaltec Aerosystems produced various metal products and disposed of wastewater containing high levels of contaminants such as trichloroethylene, tetrachloroethylene, trichloroethane, vinyl chloride, copper, and chromium in an unlined lagoon. These contaminants eventually seeped into the groundwater, affecting approximately 4,000 people who used well water.

- **Brick Township, New Jersey** - The municipal landfill accepted a variety of waste types, including septage, sewage, and chemical waste. Toxic concentrations of cadmium, lead, mercury, benzene, chlorobenzene, trichloroethane, tetrachlorethylene, and phthalates were found in the groundwater. Arsenic, cadmium, chromium, mercury, ethylbenzene, and toluene were also detected. About 3,000 people relying on well water were potentially exposed.

- **Sparta, New Jersey** - O. Polymer, a resin and plasticizer manufacturing company, contaminated the groundwater with trichloroethane, trichloroethylene, methyl isobutyl ketone, and acetone. At least 760 people, along with a park and a high school, were affected by contaminated well water.

Well, water is typically fresh, rich in nutrients, and high in minerals. It should be naturally cool and clear, with no odor.

However, vigilance is necessary to ensure its safety for drinking, bathing, and skin contact. Water systems are not regulated as public water; guidelines and legal limits have been set for more than 90 contaminants. Moving into an older home with a neglected well water system or experiencing flooding and natural disasters can create ideal conditions for bacterial growth and the accumulation of contaminants in a water supply. Some of the most concerning contaminants include:

Common Contaminants Found in Well Water

Bacteria

While bacteria are ubiquitous in nature and are usually not harmful, in some species, they can cause diseases. Pathogens can percolate through the soil and contaminate the aquifer, which is the source of the well water. These disease-causing microorganisms usually originate from animal and human waste, sewage, and stormwater. They can cause stomach pain, nausea, vomiting, diarrhea, dysentery, hepatitis, salmonellosis, giardiasis, and typhoid.

Iron

Iron is commonly found in wells. It can cause water to be discolored with a reddish-brown color and have a metallic taste. It can cause stains on bathroom fixtures such as faucets, sinks, bathtubs, and showers. Utensils washed in iron-rich water can become discolored. Over time, iron can cause pipes to become clogged.

At low levels, iron is not considered to be a health problem. However, at higher concentrations, it can result in diabetes, hemochromatosis, stomach problems, and nausea and can potentially damage the liver, pancreas, and heart.

There are three types of iron found in water. Ferrous iron is water soluble. It is not visible but may cause staining and can affect the taste of water. When ferrous-rich water is exposed to the atmosphere, it can be converted into ferric iron. Water containing ferric iron appears reddish or orange. Ferric iron is insoluble. Therefore, it can deposit on showerheads and fixtures and is responsible for clogging pipes. Bacterial iron is not harmful, but it can cause conditions where pathogens can grow and serve as a substrate for the deposition of organic compounds. The iron released by bacteria appears as a slimy red residue that can build up on home fixtures. Needless to say, iron concentrations should be minimized in both well and municipal waters. This can easily be done by passing the water through a water softener.

Arsenic

This heavy metal occurs naturally in groundwater and is also found in several pesticides. Chronic exposure to small levels of arsenic can affect child development and is toxic, especially to children. It is also known as a carcinogen. High levels of arsenic have been detected in water wells in more than 25 states, posing serious health risks such as skin cancer and skin pigmentation issues.

Cancer-Causing Agents

Chemicals like fertilizers, pesticides, and other industrial compounds seep into the ground and can leach into an aquifer used for well water, causing a risk of cancer and other adverse health effects. Compounds such as methyl tert-butyl ether (MTBE), which is used to improve fuel combustion efficiency, and vinyl chloride, found in PVC piping and packaging materials, are known carcinogens. Additionally, radioactive elements such as radium, plutonium, and uranium, which can be found in well water, can pose significant health risks and hazards when ingested over extended periods.

Nitrites

Nitrates, commonly found in soil, water, and various foods, can be converted into toxic nitrites, which can interfere with the body's ability to transport oxygen. It can cause methemoglobinemia, especially in bottle-fed babies, which can lead to death. Nitrates and nitrites may also cause an increased heart rate, nausea, headaches, and abdominal cramps. There is also some evidence that it may cause an increased risk of gastric cancer. The primary sources of nitrates and nitrites are agricultural fertilizers and animal waste.

Acidity

The pH range goes from 0 to 14, with a pH of 7 being neutral. The lower the pH, the more acidic it is. The higher the pH, the more basic or alkaline it is. The acidity of water can gradually corrode pipes, potentially causing damage and leading to the buildup of minerals in the plumbing system. This can result in hard water and a mineral buildup in faucets and pipes. To prevent this from happening, builders now use PVC pipes.

There are signs of water quality issues that can be easily observed.

Color

Healthy water should be clear and transparent. If you notice a yellowish tint, cloudiness, or discoloration, this could indicate that there are underlying water quality issues.

Odor

A distinct smell of rotten eggs, especially common in well water, may indicate high sulfur content, often caused by natural decay and chemical reactions in the surrounding soil and rock. Any distinguishable odor will indicate that the quality of the water is questionable.

Taste

Ideally, water should have no discernible taste. If you detect an off-taste, foul, or sour flavor, prudence should stop you from consuming it. By staying vigilant for these early signs and addressing any issues promptly, you can help maintain the safety and quality of the water. If the water smells bad or tastes bad, it is probably bad and should not be used.

To ensure the safety of your water supply, you should filter the water before it is used. Filters come in various forms, ranging from attachments for your faucet or refrigerator to pitchers with filters that you can keep in your refrigerator and whole-house filtration systems.

Different systems will remove different contaminants. Therefore, choose a system that targets the specific contaminants that are in your water. It's worth noting that some filters also remove fluoride, which is purposely added to municipal waters to reduce dental caries in children. Using a water filter offers peace of mind by minimizing the risks associated with compromised well water.

Home Water Treatment System

A water test will provide insight into the quality of your water and can help you determine if investing in a water filtration system is worthwhile. Further, Pharmaceuticals have been detected in water supplies even though the water meets safety standards. Thus, a water treatment system will provide an extra layer of protection.

Water testing kits are readily available online and at many home improvement centers, or you can contact water testing laboratories. Initial tests should be comprehensive so that you do not miss any toxic contaminants. The price is well worth it if it can protect your health and that of your loved ones. There are several different types of home water treatment systems, each with its own advantages and considerations:

Water Distillation

Distillation produces the purest water. However, it is not necessary to use water of this quality, as it is expensive and difficult to maintain. Distilled water does not taste very good because it does not contain any minerals, which gives it its characteristic taste. These minerals are needed by our bodies to function correctly.

Faucet And Under-Sink Systems

These systems attach directly to your faucet or are installed under the sink and have a separate water dispenser, filtering water as it flows out. They are cost-effective and easy to install, and they are used primarily to improve the taste of water by removing chlorine. This is important because chlorine can combine with other chemicals to form carcinogenic compounds. While they're an improvement over water filter pitchers, they may not offer significant benefits in improving the quality of the drinking water beyond taste and odor improvement.

Reverse Osmosis

Water purified by reverse osmosis (RO) systems is almost as pure as distilled water and is highly regarded for its effectiveness in water filtration. In these systems, water is forced through a semipermeable membrane, which removes virtually all contaminants to produce high-quality drinking water. While they require frequent membrane replacement to maintain optimal performance, RO systems excel at removing various contaminants and impurities.

This type of system should be considered for people with severe medical conditions. Under-sink purifiers are usually RO systems.

The problem with these units is that they are only useful for the faucet to which they are attached. If you have a kitchen water purifier, it does nothing to protect you when using other faucets. For example, if your bathroom faucet water is not purified, then you are using municipal or well water to brush your teeth, wash your hands and face, and shower. You are subjecting yourself to chemicals that can be absorbed through your skin, and if you use hot water, you may inhale volatile organic chemicals that are released as you wash up or bathe.

Multi-Stage Filtration Systems

A multi-stage water filtration system provides high-quality filtered water that is suitable for human consumption, even though the water quality is slightly lower than that after distillation and reverse osmosis. This usually consists of a pre-filter to remove sand and other particulates. Consider using a six-micron pre-filter because it will also reduce the concentration of bacteria. The second stage is an activated carbon filter that removes organics such as pesticides, phthalates, dioxins, and other toxic organic compounds. The third and final stage is an ion-exchange filter that removes inorganic compounds such as chlorine, divalent cations, and heavy metals such as arsenic, lead, mercury, cadmium, and chromium, which are all toxic. After the water has passed through this multi-stage treatment system, it will be of sufficiently high quality to protect your health, and the water will be so soft that there will be no scum buildup. Scum buildup on pipes and faucets occurs because the water is hard. Hard water contains divalent cations. Soft water enables a large amount of lather to be produced by a very small amount of soap.

In conclusion, distillation units are seldom used for household water needs. Reverse osmosis systems are excellent, but they are expensive to purchase and maintain. Also, the quality of the filtered water is much purer than is necessary. There is little reason to purchase an RO unit unless there are special health needs. Multi-stage filtration systems are recommended because they are moderately priced and will provide more than adequate protection. A faucet-mounted filtration system is not sufficient unless every faucet and shower has them installed. If the kitchen sink does not have a filtration system, the unfiltered water may be used for cooking or washing dishes. In the bathroom, you will not be using filtered water to brush your teeth or to shower. Showering with unfiltered water may result in the absorption of toxic chemicals through the skin into the circulatory system. Using warm, unfiltered water can result in the release of toxic Volatile Organic Chemicals, which may be inhaled. Therefore, a whole-house, multi-stage water filtration system is highly recommended.

CHAPTER 7: PREVENTING HOUSEHOLD ACCIDENTS

Accidents can happen anytime and anywhere. However, they occur most frequently in our homes. In fact, two out of three accidents happen at home. Children under the age of five and the elderly, particularly those above the age of 65, are the ones in most danger. Accidents usually occur because people either do not pay attention to what they are doing or are overtired.

According to the NSC (National Safety Council), 53.6% of all injury-involved accidents occur inside. In 2020, it was reported that 200,955 deaths occurred due to injuries encountered at home. There are more deaths resulting from household accidents than there are from motor vehicle crashes. We feel secure in our homes because it gives us comfort, solace, and a sense of security.

Accidents can range in severity from a mishap resulting in a minor bruise to severe injuries. Our homes may be our castles, but there is no guarantee that they are safe. Most of these incidents at home are avoidable, and preventative measures should be taken. The most common types of home accidents are as follows:

Falling

Falling is the number one cause of home injuries. As expected, the two groups most at risk for falls are children under the age of five and elderly adults above 65. However, everyone is subject to falling, regardless of age.

Home fixtures, such as loose carpets, slippery throw rugs, wooden flashboards that stick up, and loose electric cords, can contribute to falls, leading to back pain and other injuries. Wearing loose clothing or baggy clothes can also contribute to falls.

People slip on stairways for a variety of reasons, such as stepping on small objects left on the stairs, being slippery, losing balance, or not paying attention. Falling resulting from slipping on the stairs poses a great threat. One can sometimes slip through the staircase, even with guardrails. Serious falls can lead to concussions and death. This is why it is crucial to take precautions to prevent falls in homes.

The remedy is to keep stairs clean, lay anti-slip stair treads, make sure that stairway carpeting is not loose, ensure that the handrail does not wobble, and ensure that there is adequate lighting. Elderly individuals with limited mobility should either consider stairlifts or moving to a single-level home to prevent stairway falls.

Most importantly, to reduce the risk of accidents, pay attention to what you are doing. If you are tired, rest before you tackle a potentially dangerous task. In other words, it is wise to use common sense when danger is involved.

Bathtubs, showers, and kitchen and bathroom floors are places in the home that can become dangerous when wet. Using rubber mats in showers helps prevent falls, and placing mats or towels on the floor outside the bath or shower adds extra safety.

Elderly individuals may find hoists or shower seats beneficial for safer bathing and waterproof medical alert devices for added security.

Avoid standing on tables, chairs, or other pieces of furniture. Instead, use a ladder to reach high objects. Make sure the ladder is positioned so that it is stable. This will help to prevent unnecessary falls and injuries.

Fire Hazards

Fires pose a significant danger in households, often stemming from faulty electrical wiring, malfunctioning appliances, or even the use of candles. While some fires may be visible, they can also go unnoticed or forgotten without vigilant intervention. Over 3,000 lives are lost to fires each year in America, and it ranks as the third leading cause of home accidents.

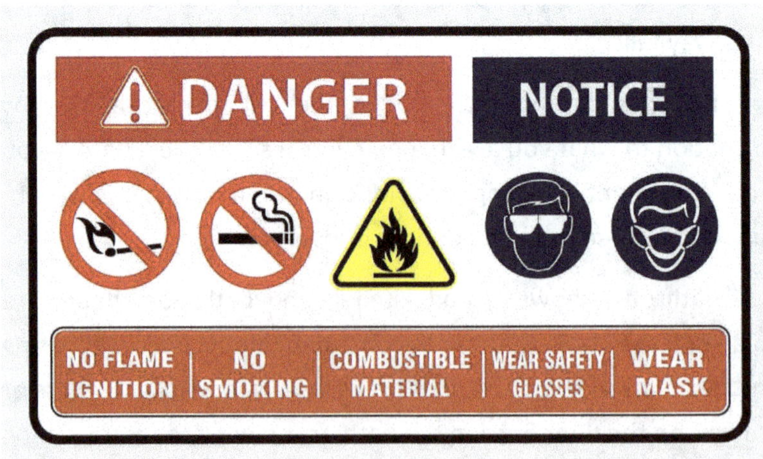
DANGER
NOTICE
NO FLAME IGNITION
NO SMOKING
COMBUSTIBLE MATERIAL
WEAR SAFETY GLASSES
WEAR MASK

The important point is to take precautions while cooking, ensuring pans of oil for deep-frying are never left unattended. If a fire occurs, use a damp cloth or a frying pan cover to smother it right away. However, never pour water on an oil fire because it will cause the fire to spread. Have electrical wiring inspected by a qualified electrician to prevent electrical fires? During the holiday season, be cautious of fire hazards, especially from faulty Christmas tree lights. Switch off all lights before bedtime or when you are going out. Keep matches and lighters away from children, carefully extinguish cigarettes, and never leave candles burning overnight. Lastly, have a fire safety plan in place that everyone in the household knows about, including an evacuation strategy.

Be sure that your home has smoke detectors. If not, install smoke detectors in key areas such as the kitchen, bedrooms, and basement, and test them monthly while replacing batteries twice a year. The best way to go is to install a home alarm system that not only alerts you to a fire but also contacts the fire department automatically in case of smoke detection. This is particularly helpful if occupants are incapacitated by smoke inhalation.

Burns And Cuts

The risk of experiencing burns or other fire-related accidents is a concern, particularly for both young children and seniors, because they have a higher likelihood of getting burned. The kitchen is especially dangerous. It is crucial to keep young children away from hot stoves or ovens to prevent burn injuries. There is also a chance someone will accidentally touch a hot oven or something that is cooking. There are other potential sources that could pose burn risks. For instance, if the water heater exceeds 120 degrees Fahrenheit, scalding can occur. There is also the threat of home fires. Turn pot handles inward, remove flammable materials, and stay close when cooking flammables like oil and fat. Every kitchen should have a fire extinguisher, and developing an emergency escape plan with the family is important to ensure everyone's safety in the event of a household fire.

Besides the potential threat of fires, badly designed or wrongly placed furniture in the home can pose a hazard. Frequently, people unintentionally bump into furniture, which can cause bruising and pain. Feet are usually the part of the body that suffers from interacting with placed furniture because they end up striking the hard furniture surfaces, leaving a person wincing in pain. Furniture drawers and closet doors can pinch fingers and hands.

Many people accidentally cut themselves while trying to slice a bagel or chop vegetables. If a knife is very sharp, there is the possibility of deep cuts that might need stitches. Using a cutting board on a non-slip surface will reduce the chances of cuts. Furthermore, the edges of opened cans can also result in cuts. Using a mechanical can opener with a magnet is a better option.

Keep kitchen knives and graters in locked drawers away from children's reach. Be sure to pay attention when you are using knives, and always remember to cut away from you. Secure razor blades in bathrooms by placing them on high shelves out of children's reach. An even better idea would be to store razor blades and other grooming tools, like cuticle scissors, in drawers with locks.

Poisoning

There are about 5,000 poison-related fatalities each year. It's especially heartbreaking because most of these incidents involve curious young children. Parents can protect their children from becoming part of these statistics by following some safety tips.

Carbon Monoxide Poisoning

Carbon monoxide is a colorless, odorless, and tasteless gas. Therefore, it usually goes undetected, and sadly, it is also one that keeps people silent. This is the reason why it is called the silent killer. It claims the lives of more than 50 people each year and sends hundreds to hospitals. However, it is important to discuss carbon monoxide poisoning in the home. Carbon monoxide levels build up in homes, especially during the winter, because there is inadequate ventilation.

When oxygen levels are lowered, carbon monoxide is produced instead of carbon dioxide. This gas can interfere with the oxygen-carrying capacity of the blood by binding with the hemoglobin in the red blood cells, resulting in anoxia. This results in headaches, fatigue, lethargy, dizziness, and drowsiness. If there is no fresh air, then there is a risk of losing consciousness and dying due to insufficient oxygen to the brain. It is one of the many common home accidents that don't usually result in death but can substantially degrade the quality of life.

Products that can produce carbon monoxide are kerosene space heaters, gas stoves, wood stoves, gas grills or ovens, charcoal, automobiles, lawnmowers, generators, or other gas-powered equipment. These are products that almost every house has. Running an automobile engine inside a closed garage can result in carbon monoxide poisoning. People should be aware of conditions that can produce carbon monoxide in their homes.

Choking

Choking is a terrifying home accident. Common hazards around homes can pose a choking hazard, especially for babies and toddlers. A crawling baby or toddler is curious about their surroundings and is continuously exploring every nook and cranny of their home, blissfully unaware of what is going into their mouths. Certain kinds of food, such as large pieces of meat or fish bones, are yet another danger, not only for toddlers but for adults too.

Choking can happen due to eating too fast, talking while chewing, or taking large bites. Children, such as toddlers, can choke on food as they are still learning how to chew properly.; hence, the risk of choking is higher in young children than in adults. This is why parental supervision during meals is important. Cutting food into small pieces is a good way to avoid choking.

A home with young children should be kept free of potential choking hazards. Small toy parts should be kept away from children under the age of 5. This includes objects such as coins, buttons, pen caps, jewelry, and coin lithium button batteries. Common gadgets, like singing cards, key fobs, thermometers, and calculators, contain small lithium-ion batteries. These batteries can become stuck in the throat, causing burns and possible death. If you are a parent of a little one, then you must store such items completely out of the children's needs. If a child swallows one of these batteries, seek emergency care right away.

Suffocation and Asphyxiation

Suffocation results from external pressure or obstruction of the respiratory airways. Various accidents can lead to this condition, such as when food or small objects become lodged in the airways, preventing the intake of air into the lungs. Older individuals who wear dentures or those who experience swallowing difficulties are more susceptible to this type of asphyxiation. Also, illnesses or injuries such as heart failure, neck fractures, or severe allergic reactions can trigger physical asphyxiation.

Asphyxiation, on the other hand, occurs when ingested substances enter the airways or lungs, often termed "going down the wrong pipe." Asphyxiation can result from oxygen deprivation in enclosed or airtight spaces. Drowning, strangulation, being smothered by an object that tightly covers the face, and when a heavy object pushes against the chest are examples of asphyxiation because they hinder the ability to breathe.

Unintentional strangulation can happen at home in many ways. Loose cords, clothing, and window blinds can be risky, especially for young children. Long strings on curtains or bedding can accidentally wrap around someone's neck. Being aware of these risks and taking steps like securing cords and watching children closely can help prevent these types of accidents.

Chemical Asphyxiation

Chemical asphyxiation occurs when a person is deprived of oxygen due to exposure to chemicals that interfere with the body's ability to use oxygen. This can potentially lead to death if not promptly addressed.

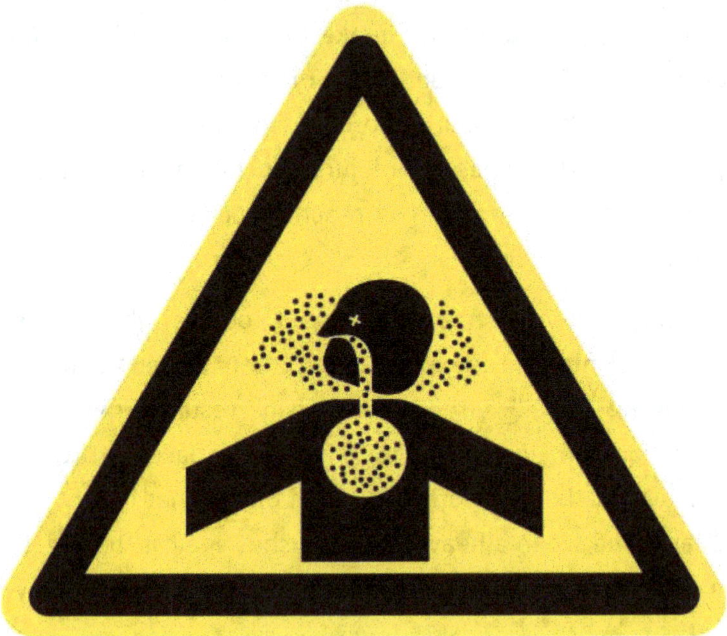

Chemical asphyxiation can occur at home through household chemicals such as bleach, ammonia, and other cleaning agents, which release toxic volatile gases when mixed or used in poorly ventilated areas. Inappropriate use or exposure to pesticides and insecticides indoors can also release toxic fumes that can impair respiratory function.

Further, chemical asphyxiation can occur through the inhalation of the Volatile Organic Compounds (VOCs) found in paints, glues, varnishes, and other solvents. Carbon monoxide is also considered to be a chemical asphyxiant. Proper ventilation, safe handling practices, and the installation of carbon monoxide detectors can help mitigate the risk of chemical asphyxiation and ensure a safer living environment.

Create A Safe Environment

Since our home is our sanctuary, we should not take it for granted when it comes to safety. It's not just children and the elderly who can get hurt; everyone is at risk. In America, home accidents claim about 18,000 lives each year and lead to 21 million medical visits, costing around $220 billion annually. Many of these accidents are preventable, and they can be life-changing events.

For families with children, child-proofing measures are important. Make sure to secure cabinets containing hazardous substances and restrict access to unsafe areas to help prevent accidents and keep children safe. Also, all cleaning agents and detergents should be kept far from the reach of children because they may be curious about these products, as their colors might attract them.

Having essential emergency supplies such as first aid kits, flashlights, and non-perishable food stocked at home should never be neglected. This ensures readiness for any unforeseen accidents or emergencies.

By taking the proper precautionary steps, not only will you feel safe at home, but you will also be safe. This should be both our desire and our ultimate goal. Feeling secure at home is important, but many people get hurt in home accidents every year, and some of these accidents are more serious than imagined. Luckily, there are ways to make homes safer and prevent accidents.

Most importantly, to reduce the risk of accidents, pay attention to what you are doing. If you are tired, rest before you tackle a potentially dangerous task. In other words, it is wise to use common sense when danger is involved. Falls and slips are common threats to anyone, and mostly stairways are a huge risk if someone falls or slips. However, they can be made safer by using anti-slip strips, checking handrail stability, and securing all carpeted areas. These measures help to prevent accidents and ensure safer navigation through the home.

CHAPTER 8: EXTERNAL DANGERS

Our backyards are places where we can relax, garden, and enjoy being outdoors. It is also a place where children can be safe while they play. However, children's play areas can pose significant dangers, so we must be proactive to minimize the risk of injury. This is important since children are not aware of potential dangers. Thus, the playground should be child-proofed to avoid accidents.

Materials like pulverized rubber, sand, wood chips, or engineered wood fiber are suitable options for safe surfacing around swing sets and playgrounds because they will cushion falls. Grassy areas can be used, but they will not provide the same level of protection from falls. Remove or cover any sharp edges or protrusions that may be found on playground equipment because they can pose a risk of cuts and bruises.

Look for uneven surfaces and holes in the lawn, as they can result in falls and broken legs. When found, even the ground and fill in the holes with a suitable material. Maintain the yard by keeping it clear of debris. Not only is debris unsightly, but people can trip over it. Also, be vigilant for tripping hazards, such as tree roots and rocks, that could lead to tripping accidents.

It is crucial to remember that minimizing outdoor safety hazards in the yard is just as important as child-proofing your home. We cannot control everything, but what we can control should not be overlooked. Another consideration in our backyard is the risk of chemical exposure. We allow our children to run around and play in the backyard safely. However, how safe is the backyard? We fertilize the grass to help it grow. We also use insecticides, fungicides, herbicides, and other types of pesticides to keep our lawns looking good. One characteristic of pesticides is that they are readily water-soluble, so they can easily spread through the lawn and be absorbed by root systems. As a result, many pesticides are easily absorbed through the skin into the circulatory system, where they can be carried to target organs. Worse, many pesticides are strong carcinogens and can cause other types of severe illnesses, especially in developing children.

As a result, children should not be permitted to play in the yard unless they are wearing shoes. It is advisable that they also wear long pants. This will minimize pesticide exposure.

Another concern is homes with swimming pools. Unfortunately, drowning is the top cause of death among young children. Therefore, they should never be left unsupervised around pools or hot tubs. The importance of a fence cannot be overstated. Safety features like fences with self-closing gates, door alarms, and pool alarms should be installed to prevent unauthorized access and to alert you if someone is in the water.

Proximity to Hazardous Sites

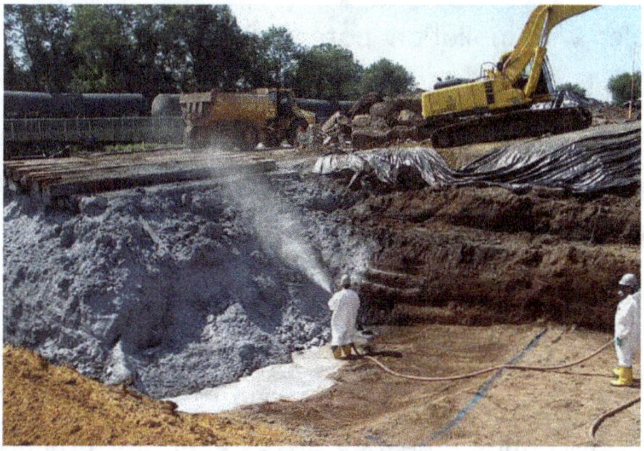

An important consideration is where your house is located in relation to hazardous waste sites, landfills, and manufacturing sites. Thus, the expression that location matters is especially true in these cases.

The proximity of a home to an industrial area or other dangerous place should be of paramount concern. Many homes are located near hazardous waste sites, manufacturing facilities, landfills, cell towers, high-power electric lines and substations, electric power plants, nuclear power plants, etc. Not only are these places aesthetically pleasing, but they can also release toxic pollutants that may contaminate the air, soil, and surface and subsurface waters. This may result in chemical exposure from any of these contaminated sources.

In chronic chemical exposures, small concentrations of toxic pollutants released over a long period of time can be an insidious hazard to a person's health. The consequences of air pollution are far-reaching, resulting in skin irritation, heart problems, respiratory issues, eye infections, cancer, and other severe illnesses. Pregnant women and their babies are particularly vulnerable, with pollution potentially causing fertility issues, miscarriages, and developmental harm to the unborn child. Furthermore, exposure to airborne toxicants can impair children's cognitive abilities, hindering their learning and development.

Industrial activities can produce noise that can harm the health and well-being of the surrounding community. Constant exposure to high noise levels can lead to various health issues, including discomfort, hearing loss, sleep disturbances, and increased levels of stress. Residents may also find it challenging to relax or engage in activities requiring concentration due to the incessant background noise emanating from a factory. Thus, noise can reduce the overall quality of life for these residents. Lack of quality sleep can have a cascading effect on overall health, contributing to fatigue, irritability, and decreased cognitive function.

Proximity to Source of Electromagnetic Radiation (EMIF)

Another concern is the proximity to sources of Electromagnetic Radiation (EMF), which are invisible energy waves. In an EMF, electric and magnetic fields join together to form a single radiation field. These can be produced by a plethora of sources, such as power lines, cell phones, microwaves, Wi-Fi routers, and computers. There is some scientific evidence that EMFs may adversely affect human health.

There are two types of EMFs. High-frequency EMFs are high-energy rays that can be emitted by medical equipment like X-ray machines and CT scans, as well as by sources like gamma radiation from radioactive elements such as uranium, plutonium, and radon and UV radiation from the sun and tanning beds. These high-energy rays are considered to be ionizing radiation and have been found to be able to damage cells and their chromosomes. Exposure to high levels of high-frequency EMFs can harm human DNA and cells, but the likelihood of encountering such high levels in your daily life is very low. Also, exposure, if it occurs, usually occurs in small amounts. Luckily, this type of EMF is not commonly found in homes.

The second type of EMF is low-frequency EMF, classified as non-ionizing radiation. Non-ionizing EMFs originate from both natural and man-made sources. The earth's magnetic field is an example of a natural EMF. Man-made Low-frequency electromagnetic Radiation fields are produced by cell towers, high-power electric lines, and electric substations. These EMFs can also come from everyday household appliances such as microwave ovens, cellphones, hair dryers, washing machines, electric shavers, and electric blankets. Another type of non-ionizing radiofrequency radiation, extremely low-frequency EMFs (ELF-EMFs), emanates from wireless devices such as cell phones, smart meters, tablets, and laptops, as well as from radio and television signals, radar, satellite stations, and MRI machines.

It has been shown to adversely affect the nervous system and brain cognitive function. These fields have also been shown to result in increased levels of skin cancer as well. However, there is insufficient evidence to determine if it can cause brain cancer or other types of tumors. Although this form of EMF is considered by some scientists to pose little danger to human health, there is existing evidence that there may be an increased danger to the nervous system and to brain cognitive function resulting from chronic exposure. As with all types of exposures, the amount of exposure and the length of exposure are the two biggest concerns.

Although every electrical device in the home emits EMFs, most people's exposure to EMFs is very low. When you're close to appliances like refrigerators, microwaves, and washing machines, you might experience short-term high exposures to EMF radiation, but exposure levels decrease rapidly as you move away from them. You can use an EMF meter to check EMF levels in your home, which you can easily buy online. Ask your local power company for an on-site reading.

Electromagnetic force levels can vary within a home. Therefore, be sure to test different areas to get a more accurate picture of the exposure risks. Also, check readings at various points on your walls since electric wires may be behind the walls. If you find high EMF readings near your bed, consider relocating it to a different area with lower levels.

Using your cell phone and household appliances, including power lines, should be safe. The strength of EMFs generated by appliances rapidly decreases with distance. At a distance of one foot, the magnetic fields from most household appliances are more than 100 times weaker than the source. So, avoid sitting or staying close to appliances for too long. While you might need to close the door to turn on the TV or microwave, take a few steps away after you have turned them on. Do not keep a cell phone next to your bed when you sleep. Instead, put it a couple of feet away so that it is easily accessible but will not be an inherent danger. Consider using the speaker function or earbuds when talking on the phone to reduce the amount of RF exposure to your brain. Earpieces emit a lower power of EMF than our cell phones.

The salient question is how far a house should be from a dangerous facility in order to be considered safe. This is speculative because there are no specific guidelines to refer to. Thus, it is better to exercise an abundance of caution when considering this question. In most cases, a half-mile from an industrial facility or a site that can produce electromagnetic radiation should be sufficient. However, if there is a large manufacturing or petrochemical plant, then living at least a mile from the site would be a more prudent distance due to the potential release of high levels of airborne toxicants. Regarding nuclear power plants, the further away you can live from them, the safer you will be. This will minimize your exposure in the case of a nuclear meltdown and to the accidental release of radioactive gases.

CHAPTER 9: HOUSEHOLD HEALTH

Buying a house is one of the biggest decisions of your life. It is not just limited to paying it off, getting it furnished well, and decorating it. There are many steps along the complex way to ownership, and the road can be a bit bumpy. Numerous things come together, including meeting important deadlines and involving multiple parties, to make the process steady and successful. There are crucial steps to take when buying a home.

Homes should provide the safest place where we can find comfort, protection, and safety. Hence, it is crucial to be sure that there are no threats or hazards hidden in or around the home that can potentially cause you harm. Have the house inspected, not only looking at the structure but also paying attention to potential environmental issues that could plague you in the future. It might be tempting to purchase a new home with a steady process and move in right away after signing the deal but *don't rush.* Instead, thoroughly inspect the house to avoid dealing with issues in the future, which might turn your excitement about buying a new home into a bitter experience. These issues may create a great deal of stress trying to remediate them, and they may also be costly.

Foundation And Structural Cracks

When you're buying a home, cracks in the walls are more than just a cosmetic issue. Depending on their size, they can indicate problems with the property's foundation and pose both security and health risks. Cracks in the foundation can allow moisture, insects, and rodent pests into the home. Thus, it is essential to investigate the foundation for any problems. Cracks in the walls and ceiling are often the most visible. If there's no basement, inspect the doors—are they easy to close?—and see if the door frames are square and consistent in size. If anything seems off, consider it a warning sign that there are problems with the foundation.

Poor Drainage

Another key aspect to consider for home safety is the quality of drainage. Excess moisture or standing water next to the side of the house is a sign of poor drainage. Look for stains on the walls, especially in the basement. Addressing a problem with poor drainage will lessen the chance of mold and mildew growing in the house. Being attentive to these details during your home inspection can prevent potential in-home security issues once you've settled into your new property.

Outdated Electrical Systems

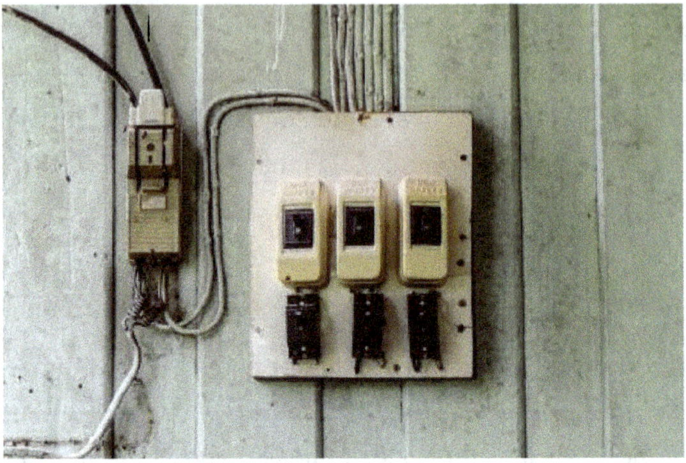

Outdated electrical systems in the house are a potential safety hazard. Not only is old wiring a potential hazard, but it can also affect your ability to get homeowners insurance. The electrical demands of today were not anticipated in the past, and thus, the system may not be able to carry the electrical load. As a result, frequent circuit overloads and disruptions may occur. Safety standards are more stringent than they were in the past, so an older electrical system may not comply with modern safety standards. This may lead to electric hazards such as fires or electrical shocks.

Proper Ventilation

Good air circulation keeps a house fresh. When air can circulate freely, it prevents hot air from getting trapped indoors, helping to keep the room temperature a few degrees cooler. If the home is not ventilated properly, airborne pollutants such as mold, pet dander, mites, bacteria, and fungus can accumulate, increasing the risk of asthma and other health problems.

Even if the quality of air outside is not very good, the air quality in a sealed home is worse. Pollutants tend to be more concentrated indoors due to limited space and a lack of adequate air circulation. This means that you breathe in a larger concentration of airborne pollutants with each breath compared to being outside.

Climate

Climate change is causing an increase in the number of natural disasters. Not only are these disasters becoming more frequent, but they are also becoming more severe. The potential for these disasters poses a real set of challenges for homeowners.

Climate risks are increasingly playing a major role in influencing the decision to buy a home. Wildfires, coastal erosion, and heavy rains affected properties from Greece to Italy and throughout the United States.

Homebuyers are becoming concerned if the homes they are considering are even worth it. There is an increasing concern about flooding, hurricanes, tornadoes, extreme heat, wildfires, and other climate-related hazards. Therefore, you must strategically plan to minimize the effects of these potential natural disasters and protect your home. If a home is damaged, it can open the door to many hazards and subsequent health issues.

Housing Affects Health

Most Americans spend roughly 90 percent of their time indoors, with about two-thirds of that time spent at home. This is especially true for young children, who are particularly vulnerable to hazards within the household. Housing-related factors can greatly impact our health, either positively or negatively. There are three key aspects of housing and their connections to health: the physical conditions inside homes, the conditions of the surrounding neighborhood, and housing affordability. These factors not only influence the quality of homes and neighborhoods but also affect families' ability to make healthy choices overall.

Having a healthy home is important for both physical and mental well-being. A safe and hazard-free home is essential for good health. On the other hand, poor quality or inadequate housing can lead to health issues like chronic diseases and injuries and can even affect childhood development. Homes often have multiple hazards, like poor indoor air quality and lead paint, putting families at risk for various health problems. For instance:

Lead poisoning can harm a child's brain development, leading to lower intelligence and reading difficulties.

Substandard housing, such as leaks, poor ventilation, and pests, can increase mold and allergens, affecting health.

Cold indoor temperatures have been linked to cardiovascular issues, while high temperatures can increase mortality, especially among the elderly.

Crowded living conditions have been associated with physical illnesses such as tuberculosis and respiratory infections, as well as psychological distress in both adults and children.

The neighborhood where a home is located can greatly impact health and the conditions inside a home. A neighborhood's social, physical, and economic characteristics significantly affect short- and long-term health and longevity.

Neighborhoods with positive attributes, including safe places for children to play and for adults to exercise free from crime, violence, and pollution, promote health. Access to grocery stores offering fresh produce and fewer fast-food outlets can make it easier for families to eat wholesome meals. Additionally, neighborhoods with good social and economic conditions provide greater access to job opportunities, efficient transportation, and quality public resources such as police services and schools. However, not all neighborhoods have these advantages, and access to health-promoting conditions varies depending on household economic and social resources. The concentration of poor-quality housing in less advantaged neighborhoods exacerbates racial, ethnic, and socioeconomic disparities in health.

According to the World Health Organization (WHO), the quality of housing has a major impact on health. Poor housing is related to a wide range of health conditions, such as respiratory diseases, including asthma, cardiovascular diseases, injuries, mental health, infectious diseases, tuberculosis, influence, and diarrhea. Therefore, housing has become an important issue in public health.

When we talk about health, we often focus on things like exercise, diet, and outdoor pollution. However, we tend to overlook the importance of the air we breathe indoors. If the air indoors is of poor quality, it can seriously affect our health, causing various issues that need attention.

Inhaling airborne pollutants, whether for a short or long time, can cause many diseases. These include stroke, chronic obstructive pulmonary disease (COPD), and various cancers like those of the trachea, bronchus, and lungs. Air pollution can also make asthma worse and increase the risk of both upper and lower respiratory infections.

According to the World Health Organization (WHO), air pollution is linked to conditions including type 2 diabetes, obesity, inflammation, Alzheimer's disease, and dementia. The International Agency for Research on Cancer has even classified air pollution, especially PM2.5, as a major cause of cancer.

A review by the Forum of International Societies Environmental Committee states that long-term exposure to air pollution can affect every part of the body, aggravating existing health problems. Factors that make indoor air quality worse include not having enough ventilation, which allows pollutants to build up. Other factors include allergens, irritants, and the use of chemical cleaning products. Even everyday activities such as cooking and smoking can contribute to poor indoor air quality. Also, improperly maintained HVAC systems and mold or dampness can worsen indoor air pollution. Finding and fixing these problems is important to keep the quality of interior air at acceptable levels.

Allergies and Asthma Triggers

Indoor environments contain various allergens that can provoke allergic reactions. Common indoor allergens include dust mites, pet dander, mold spores, and cockroach debris. These allergens can lead to symptoms like sneezing, itching, watery eyes, and congestion, particularly in sensitive individuals.

Poor indoor air quality worsens the symptoms of allergies and asthma. Exposure to indoor allergens can trigger asthma attacks and intensify allergic reactions. People with allergies or asthma should take the location of the house into consideration to minimize the potential for exposure to allergens.

Unhygienic Conditions

Homes can vary in their cleanliness, corresponding to the differences in people. Many people keep their houses orderly and spotless, although most do not go to these extremes. However, they keep their houses relatively clean. However, there are others who are not overly concerned about the cleanliness of their homes, which can result in poor sanitation and unhygienic conditions. This can lead to the spread of illnesses and infections, as well as increase the likelihood of exposure to allergens. Therefore, houses should be kept as clean as possible to minimize the occupant's potential for exposure to bacterial and viral pathogens, suspended particulates, mold and mildew, and the presence of allergens. The cleanliness of a house can be improved if people remove their shoes when they enter the house. This will minimize carrying dirt and pollutants into the home.

Chemical Exposures

Indoor environments can contain harmful chemicals that pose health risks. These chemicals are commonly found in cleaning products, building materials, furniture, and air fresheners. Examples include formaldehyde, benzene, and Volatile Organic Compounds (VOCs). Chronic exposure to these chemicals can result in both short-term and long-term health effects. Exposure to indoor toxic chemicals can result in various health issues.

Short-term effects may include headaches, dizziness, and irritation of the eyes, nose, and throat. Long-term exposure can be more severe, potentially leading to respiratory problems, neurological disorders, and certain types of cancer. It's essential to minimize exposure to these chemicals to safeguard your health.

Cardiovascular Diseases

An often-overlooked aspect of poor air quality is that it can have a profound impact on our cardiovascular system. We usually think about outdoor air pollution when it comes to heart health risks. However, indoor air quality can also affect our heart health significantly.

Indoor air pollution, caused by things like tobacco smoke, Volatile Organic Compounds (VOCs), and suspended particulates, can increase the risk of developing cardiovascular diseases.

Indoor air pollutants can cause inflammation, oxidative stress, and problems with blood vessel function, all of which contribute to cardiovascular diseases. Studies have shown that poor indoor air quality is linked to a higher risk of heart attacks, strokes, and high blood pressure.

Poor Lighting

Often, people will keep turning off all unnecessary lights in the house as a cost-saving measure. However, the house should be properly lit to maximize our health. Inadequate lighting can lead to eye strain and fatigue, headaches and migraines, and an increased risk of falls and accidents. Additionally, it can cause Seasonal Affective Disorder (SAD). This is a type of depression that most often occurs in the Fall and Winter when the days are shorter. However, it can also occur when the interior provides minimal light. As a result, it is better to spend a bit more on lighting. The cost should be minimally different due to the common use of LED light bulbs. These bulbs come in different shades to maximize their effect on a particular room.

Noise Pollution

One reason that the location of a house is important is because of the potential for excessive noise. There is always going to be a certain amount of ambient noise coming from within and outside of the home. However, elevated noise levels can come from a myriad of sources, including airplanes flying over the house, railroad trains passing by, loud neighbors, and appliances such as steam radiators or air conditioning units. Prolonged exposure to noise pollution can result in stress and anxiety, sleep disturbances, and hearing loss resulting from long-term exposures, and it can result in cardiovascular problems such as hypertension and heart disease. This should be considered before you purchase a new home.

Mental Well-Being

The air we breathe can impact our mental health. If indoor air quality is poor and contains high levels of pollutants and allergens, it can make us feel more anxious, depressed, or have trouble thinking clearly. Breathing in air contaminated with mold, strong chemicals, or carbon monoxide can affect how our brain works and how we feel overall. Living or working in a place with bad ventilation, high humidity, or strong smells can also affect our mood and our ability to focus. These conditions can make us more irritable, cause trouble concentrating, and make us less productive.

How To Mitigate Health Risks

There are strategies that can be implemented to improve indoor air quality and reduce the risk of inhaling bad air. As discussed previously, the location of the house certainly matters. Since we know what to look for in a house before it is purchased, it is crucial to keep the home fresh, tidy, and clean. It is the duty of all of the occupants of a home to be vigilant for possible threats in the house.

"Your home should be a sanctuary for your health."

Toxic pollutants, particulates, and microorganisms can build up in your home and become a risk to your health. Therefore, do not neglect house cleaning. House dust comes from numerous sources, 60% of which originate from the immediate outdoor environment. The remaining 40% comes from indoor sources such as fibers from clothes, carpets, furnishings, cleaning products, skin, and hair. These contaminants threaten health as dust carries microplastics, persistent organic pollutants, perfluorinated chemicals, trace metals, and bacterial communities.

The level of risk depends on the amount of the contaminant you're exposed to, its toxicity level, and the duration of exposure. Children under five are at the highest risk because they are small, closer to the ground, and often put their hands in their mouths, which increases their intake of contaminants.

Identifying Common Indoor Air Pollutants

Understanding and dealing with common indoor air pollutants is vital for making indoor air healthier. These pollutants include mold, dust mites, pet dander, smoke, VOCs, and particulates. By knowing where these pollutants come from and taking steps to reduce them, the air breathed indoors will be much safer.

Implementing Proper Ventilation Systems

The use of ventilation systems cannot be stressed enough. This is key to keeping indoor air clean. Good ventilation eliminates stale air and brings in fresh air. Using exhaust fans or mechanical ventilation circulates air, thus preventing the buildup of indoor pollutants that can result in adverse health effects. This should be considered when inspecting a house to purchase. The number of windows, whether all of them are open, and how much sunlight falls on the house are further considerations. Additionally, proper ventilation keeps the house's temperature moderate.

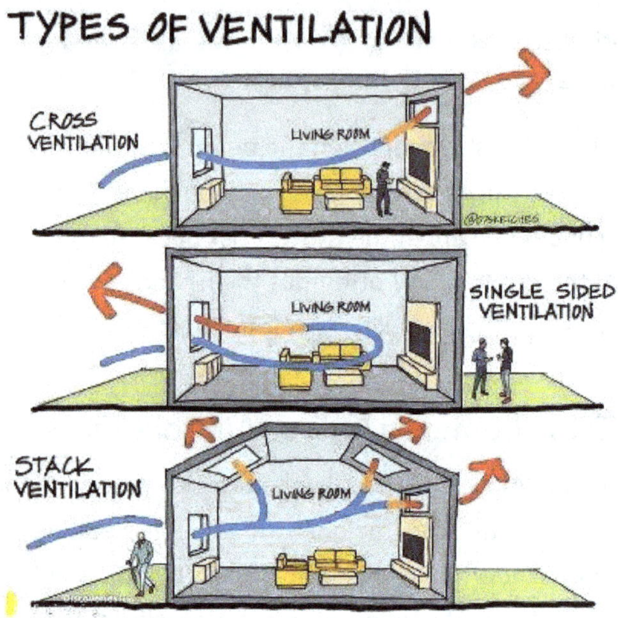

Regular Cleaning

Regular cleaning and maintenance are crucial for decreasing indoor air pollutants. Dusting, vacuuming, and mopping surfaces help eliminate allergens, dust, and other particles that affect air quality. Also, inspecting and maintaining HVAC systems can prevent the accumulation of mold, dust, and other contaminants, which can then be circulated throughout the area.

Using a vacuum with a HEPA filter will help get rid of contaminants. Get rid of household items and avoid décor that can harbor health-associated issues. For instance, shower curtains emit VOCs (Volatile Organic Compounds), and plastic leach phthalates (semi-Volatile Organic Compounds).

Air Filters And House Plants

Using air purifiers and indoor plants is another way to enhance indoor air quality. Air purifiers work by filtering out dust, smoke, pollen, and other particles, making the air cleaner to breathe. Also, indoor plants can naturally purify the air by absorbing certain toxins, removing carbon dioxide, and releasing oxygen. Plants like snake plants, spider plants, and peace lilies are especially effective for this purpose.

Be sure to use the right tools and strategies to keep your house healthy and clean, as your house's health is your health.

CHAPTER 10: HOME ENVIRONMENT AND MENTAL WELL-BEING

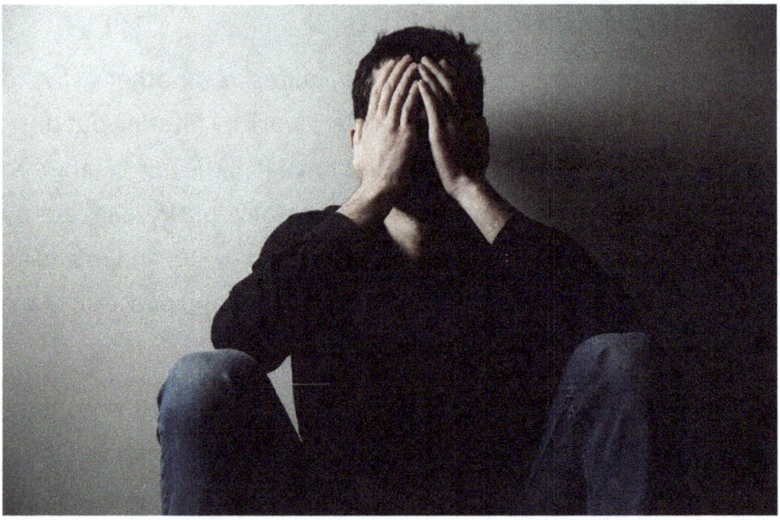

Just taking a proper bath and putting on fresh clothes makes us feel better; the same goes for keeping the house tidy. A clean and well-kept place positively affects us. Have you ever noticed the effect of the environment on your mood? Our living space is intrinsically connected to our mental health, including the places where we spend most of our time, like schools or workplaces. These places are considered environmental factors for mental well-being.

How an environment can breed mold and fungus has been previously discussed. Dust allergens and exposure to toxins affect indoor air quality, leading to physical difficulties such as respiratory and cardiovascular diseases. Our surroundings influence our moods. An adequately clean and well-maintained environment is pleasing to the eyes and gives off good vibes overall. However, our environment is not limited only to visuals.

We tend to spend most of our time in our favorite spots at home. When we spend a lot of time in a particular area, we cease to notice what's really around us. The piles of paperwork on the home computer desk and the laundry spilling out of the closet seem to disappear when we stop paying attention to them. This phenomenon is known as habituation, also called attentional blindness. The pile of laundry waiting to be washed and the clutter scattered on your desk are still there, sitting for days and even weeks. You simply do not notice them anymore or pay attention to them because you are not consciously focusing on your surroundings. Seemingly, the clutter or mess is harmless, but it is gradually taking a toll on our mental health.

The unique odors in our room, the temperature, the lighting, and the sounds around us are just as important as what we see; they all affect how we feel. These factors matter, especially for young adults who spend hours each day staring at screens for work, classes, or recreation.

Depression and Stress Are Linked to Environmental Factors

Our surroundings shape our mood, whether we live in the city or the countryside, with family or roommates, in a new building or an old house. Our mood can also affect our space; for example, when we're feeling down, we might not have the energy to tidy up or let in fresh air and light. It's a cycle that can worsen mental health.

It is crucial to break this vicious cycle before it leads to a major decline, which can further exacerbate the situation. Environmental factors that impact our mental health may intertwine with other issues. For example, depression might lead to unemployment, which can then result in poverty, inadequate nutrition, and other environmental challenges. Similarly, mental health conditions like hoarding can contribute to environmental issues, creating a harmful cycle.

Clutter can make you stressed. When we see that our rooms are messy and everything is scattered, we can become exhausted just by the sight of it. Clutter and mess can cause stress and anxiety and even lead to feelings of rage, negatively impacting our well-being.

Thus, clutter is linked to stress and anxiety. Almost everything about how we feel boils down to perception and brain signaling. When we see a cluttered home, a signal is sent to our brain that work isn't done. We become anxious because we feel overwhelmed by it.

A cluttered space overwhelms our senses, diverting our focus from what's truly important and causing stress. It draws our attention away from where it ought to be, making it difficult to relax physically and mentally. The constant reminder of unfinished tasks in a cluttered environment adds to our anxiety, leaving us unsure about how much effort it will take to restore order. Clutter also evokes feelings of embarrassment and guilt, hindering productivity and making it challenging to locate items when needed.

However, nothing in this world is insurmountable. The good news is that addressing one issue often helps with another. There will always be time to declutter your space to combat anxiety and stress. Many of us are inherently lazy or have crammed schedules that prevent us from cleaning and organizing our living space. Thus, the brain continues to receive signals of unattended work, which contributes to anxiety.

If you are unable to resolve the situation on your own for any reason, don't hesitate to seek help. You can ask your friends and family or even hire professional organizers to assist you. This should undoubtedly improve your well-being.

The Psychological Impact of Clutter

As stated, clutter can have a deep, detrimental effect on our mental well-being and overall quality of life. We must examine the sources of clutter and how remaining unkempt can specifically impact our well-being. Decluttering helps restore peace of mind, and the psychology behind it is not complex.

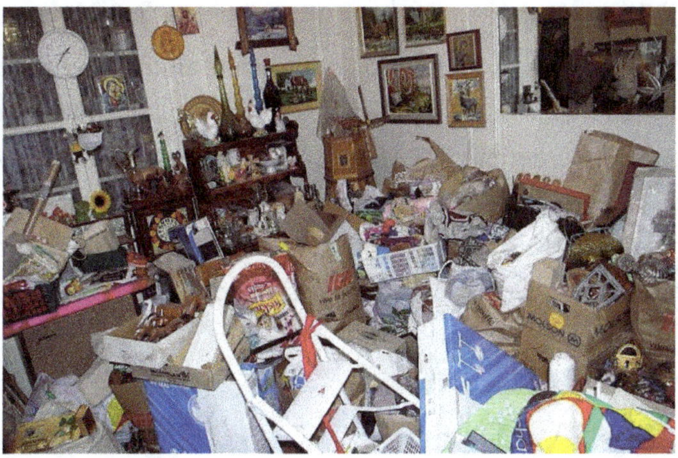

Clutter Is Linked to Stress

A cluttered environment can result in psychological distress. A disorderly space may negatively impact the brain. A study by Princeton University found that clutter—whether physical or digital—competes for a person's attention. This competition decreases task performance and increases levels of the stress hormone cortisol.

Clutter Overloads the Senses

Clutter may have a cumulative effect on the brain. The more we are exposed to clutter, the more distracted we become, causing us to lose focus and work less efficiently.

Our brains are designed to incline towards order over chaos. If our surroundings are messy and scattered, our brains are more likely to become fatigued, resulting in poor focus.

Additionally, this visual distraction from physical or digital clutter increases cognitive overload and may diminish working memory.

Factors such as health problems, financial struggles, a lack of organizational skills, ADHD, and past trauma can contribute to messiness. Sometimes, clutter is a visual sign of deeper issues, such as perfectionism. Feelings of shame, self-criticism, and comparing oneself to others, along with deeply held beliefs about creativity and messiness, can also play a role.

The Psychology Behind Hoarding

Messy spaces do not always indicate that a person is lazy, nor do they necessarily reflect moral failures or fundamental character flaws. Emotional attachment to possessions can lead to clutter. For some, these objects carry sentimental value, but excessive attachment can result in disorder.

Hoarding is often accompanied by anxiety and can lead to depression. Studies using brain scans have found similar patterns in hoarders, including strong emotional connections to objects and intense anxiety about making decisions. While hoarding may ease anxiety, it can also exacerbate it. As hoarders accumulate more items, they may feel safer from the world's dangers. However, this isolation grows, distancing them from family and friends. Even thinking about getting rid of hoarded items can provoke extreme panic and discomfort.

The only solution is to develop awareness of attachment patterns and let go of items that are no longer necessary, as "less is more." This behavior can encourage hoarders to value experiences over material possessions.

Indoor Air Quality and Mental Health

The link between air quality and mental health is often overlooked. Research indicates that "healthy air is essential for healthy minds." As discussed in previous chapters, outdoor air pollution significantly impacts our physical health. However, the effects of poor indoor air quality on our mental well-being should also be considered.

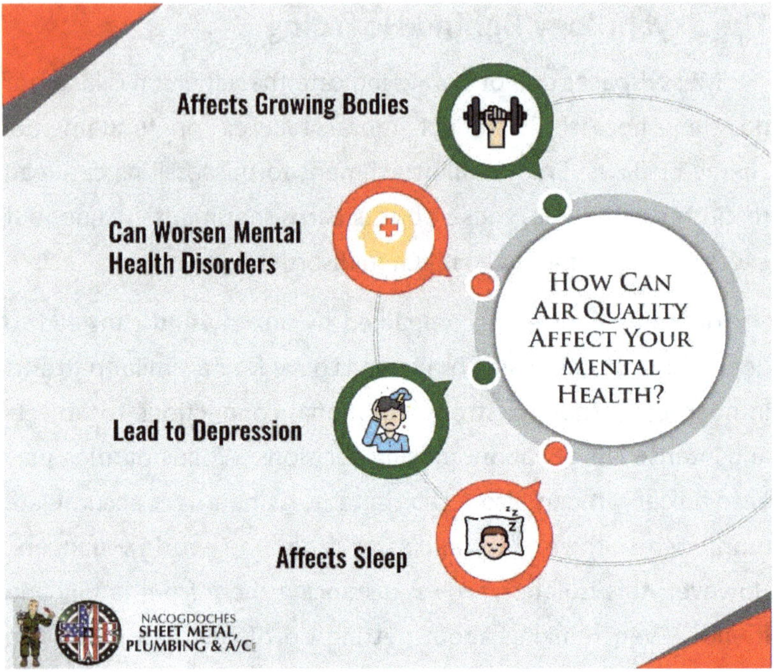

In general, many people are not aware of the relationship between contaminated indoor air and mental health. Poor air quality not only indicates a reduced quality of life but also poses risks to one's mental well-being. In fact, the World Health Organization has indicated that virtually everyone is exposed to unsafe levels of air pollution.

For example, inadequate oxygen levels can lead to issues such as depression, which, in severe cases, may escalate to suicidal thoughts. In a report for the World Economic Forum, Dr. Clara G. Zundel, the study's lead author, noted that exposure to polluted air can lead to changes in brain regions that regulate emotions. As a result, individuals breathing polluted air may face a heightened risk of anxiety and depression compared to those who breathe cleaner air. Additionally, unhealthy air has been linked to symptoms of anxiety. Living in areas with high levels of airborne toxins may also contribute to the development of neurological conditions like dementia, Alzheimer's disease, and Parkinson's disease. Children are particularly vulnerable because their brains are still developing. The World Health Organization estimates that nearly 99% of the entire population is exposed to unsafe levels of air pollution.

Airborne particulates and other toxic pollutants in households can inflame the respiratory airways and lungs, impair the immune response, and reduce the oxygen-carrying capacity of blood. Small particulates, such as PM 2.5, have been strongly associated with brain damage because they can pass through the barriers of the lungs and enter brain tissue through the olfactory nerve, damaging the cerebral blood vessels and brain nerves.

As previously stated, prolonged exposure to low levels of toxic substances can lead to insidious changes in a person's health. Likewise, slow alterations in mental health may result from chronic exposure to indoor pollutants. Thus, indoor air pollution should be considered a potential cause for changes in behavior and alterations in a person's mental health.

Tidy Home, Happy Life

As the saying goes, home is where the heart is. Our home is a place that provides comfort and meaningful memories, truly reflecting who we are, not just what's trendy. Hence, it is crucial to keep this place beautiful. However, "beautiful" doesn't necessarily mean lavish and luxurious. A beautiful home is one where we can be happy, make memories, and feel comfortable.

A beautiful home can also mean one that is well-kept and taken care of, adorned with things you love. Home and health go hand in hand; your space is linked to your mental well-being, and it must never be neglected. There are strategies to make your house the perfect home for you.

Declutter for Mental Well-Being

On the bright side, decluttering has been proven to improve mental health and overall well-being. Sorting through your belongings, getting rid of what you don't need, and organizing what's left can make you feel better both immediately and in the long run.

Decluttering isn't just about making space; it also gives you a sense of control and accomplishment. It can help you feel more confident and in charge of your life. Additionally, focusing on decluttering can help distract you from feelings of anxiety or restlessness. Another advantage is that cleaning involves physical activity, which can boost your mood by releasing endorphins.

Cleaning Can Be Therapeutic

Engaging in cleaning tasks like folding, wiping, and sorting can have similar benefits to counseling or meditation. These activities help activate the calming part of your nervous system, which can be especially helpful when you're feeling stressed.

You can also clear your mind and emotions by intentionally dealing with clutter. Transforming messy areas into tidy spaces can make you feel accomplished and boost your confidence. It also creates a physical environment that supports ongoing progress. Moreover, clearing away physical clutter can open up space for emotional reflection or letting go of negative energies. Therapists have recognized the emotional healing potential of cleaning activities.

Mindfulness and a Tidy Environment: The Best Duo

Creating tidy spaces aligns with mindfulness practices by reflecting desired internal states of mental organization and external clarity. When your surroundings are orderly, it sends signals to your nervous system that everything is okay, fostering a sense of safety and grounding. This sets the stage for other mindful activities like meditation, reflection, or creative visualization.

Engaging in regular tidying tasks also promotes a meditative state by quieting mental chatter and focusing your awareness on the present moment. Whether you're wiping, folding, or sorting, you become fully immersed in the action, making conscious decisions about what to keep and what to let go of. Purposefully using your senses in these tasks helps to calm your mind and bring clarity to your thoughts.

Creating Comfort

Making your living space mentally healthy provides comfort, support, and a sense of calm. You can achieve this by surrounding yourself with items that bring you comfort—like your favorite blanket, meaningful gifts, or candles with soothing scents. Additionally, your home's colors, natural light, and layout can influence your mental well-being. By choosing appropriate lighting, furniture textures, and room organization, you can help alleviate symptoms of anxiety and depression.

Monitor Air Quality

Ensuring good air quality can enhance oxygen levels in your brain, improving mood and concentration. It also helps lower stress hormone levels and promote better sleep. While breathing fresh outdoor air is ideal due to its additional natural benefits, filtered air can also safeguard your well-being. Similarly, various breathing techniques offer similar advantages.

Exposure to polluted outdoor air affects the brain, impacting mental health and brain function. Increased symptoms and behaviors related to mental health challenges have been observed among those exposed to high levels of air pollution. Many studies exploring different breath awareness and regulation methods have shown effectiveness in reducing stress, depression, and symptoms of PTSD.

Choosing Minimalism

After decluttering, it is crucial to resist the urge to accumulate more things for the sake of your home, yourself, and the environment. Minimalist designs embrace the principle of "less is more," avoiding clutter and creating a timeless home that's easy to maintain.

Scandinavian minimalism takes a gentle approach, prioritizing comfort, or "hygge," which suggests warmth and coziness. This style incorporates organic, eco-friendly materials like hemp rugs, woven baskets, curved wooden chairs, and ceramics in natural and white glazes rather than stainless steel, chrome, and lacquered plastics commonly found in traditional minimalism.

Scandinavian minimalism emphasizes simplicity and practicality in the home, focusing on quality over quantity. It encourages the gradual curation of your home, prioritizing quality pieces that serve a purpose and will stand the test of time.

Lighting

When illuminating your interior space, consider using both natural sunlight and indoor lighting to create an invigorating and comforting ambiance. Natural light offers a plethora of health benefits, from boosting your vitamin D levels to warding off seasonal blues and enhancing sleep quality. The simplest way to maximize natural light is cost-free: just ensure your windows aren't obstructed. Experiment with furniture arrangements or swap heavy drapes for airy voiles. Create a sunny reading nook next to a window.

Indoor lighting plays a pivotal role in setting the mood. It can completely transform a space, infusing it with warmth, opulence, and a cozy vibe. While investing in new light fixtures may seem daunting, the payoff is undeniable.

The Color of the Room

The field of color psychology operates on the premise that mere exposure to certain colors can yield tangible results, such as surrounding oneself with orange hues to boost energy levels. According to the principles of color theory, emotional issues can be alleviated by the influence of colors. This is referred to as chromotherapy or color healing. Color theory proposes that distinct colors and their corresponding frequencies can have both physiological and psychological effects on one's moods and actions.

For instance, individuals experiencing stress or anger might opt for exposure to the color blue to attain a calm state and reduce their heart rate. Similarly, individuals grappling with depression may find solace in shades of red and yellow, as these hues can augment their energy levels.

A Basic Guide to Colors

Bright, warm colors (reds, oranges, and yellows) bring energy and happiness, while cool, subdued colors (blues, greens, and purples) have a calming effect. Use bright, warm colors in entertaining areas like dining rooms and kitchens, and opt for cool colors in relaxing spaces like bedrooms and bathrooms.

Interacting More with Nature

Nature can have a significant effect on our physical and mental well-being. Spending time outdoors can effectively diminish stress levels while enhancing mood and self-esteem. We need not relocate to a natural paradise, as there are numerous methods to incorporate nature into our living space. Introducing houseplants, taking outdoor strolls, or integrating natural elements such as bamboo into your decor all offer avenues to embrace nature. Displaying a photograph or painting depicting a scenic landscape can also significantly uplift the spirits.

One good idea is to designate a stress-free area within the home—whether it's a room, a corner in the living room, or even a garden shed. Personalize the space with items like plants, candles, cherished photos, or cozy furnishings that bring you joy. Use this area for relaxing activities such as reading, napping, meditating, or simply unwinding. Every home should have a designated stress-free zone for moments when life becomes overwhelming, enabling us to achieve a better quality of life.

CHAPTER 11: TYING IT ALL TOGETHER

Safety is crucial because it reduces the possibility of accidents, whether they occur outside, at the workplace, or at home. Throughout this book, emphasis has been placed on how we can minimize household threats. Some threats escape our attention due to a lack of awareness; however, these problems can pose a silent risk to us and our families. This book aims to make readers aware of the root causes of many health issues, such as allergies, chronic diseases, and disturbed mental health, which may stem from our home or workplace—where we spend most of our time. While this may not be true for everyone, unfortunately, it is often the case.

Implementing safety rules and addressing potential problems can save us much grief. It takes commitment, careful planning, and diligence.

Indoor Pollutants

Indoor pollutants include asbestos, biological pollutants, carbon monoxide (CO), lead, pesticides, radon, Volatile Organic Compounds (VOCs), and indoor particulate matter. All of these pollutants can threaten our physical and mental well-being.

Biological threats, such as dust mites, can be our worst enemies because they can cause various health problems. Toxins in pesticides, cleaning agents, and other chemicals can lead to respiratory issues when there is chronic exposure to these substances.

The air we breathe in a closed environment essentially comes from the outdoors. However, over time, it becomes more polluted than outdoor air because it is trapped within an enclosure, and the air quality decreases as it circulates. This is why proper ventilation is so important.

Particulate matter is one of the leading causes of severe diseases, such as allergies, asthma, and lung cancer. Fine particulates, including PM 2.5, are particularly harmful if they persist at high levels, as this can double the risk of health problems like heart disease, asthma, and low birth weight.

Our homes are prone to invisible threats such as carbon monoxide—known as the silent killer—dust particles, lead dust, leaky roofs, and damp areas harboring fungus and mold. These can create an unpleasant environment that is unsuitable for living.

These household hazards are often insidious, causing an imperceptible decline in our health. While the world outside our home may be polluted, indoor air is usually worse, triggering allergies and breathing problems that can affect our overall well-being. Unacceptable levels of air pollution may be found in the homes of people living in neglected neighborhoods or near industrial areas.

It is not expected to be found in affluent suburban areas; however, both types of areas have been shown to experience elevated levels of indoor air pollution. Thus, homeowners do not typically consider indoor air pollution a serious concern. When the air is bad, health suffers, and when health suffers, it is difficult for a person to feel happy and relaxed. A healthy environment should be considered a form of wealth because we depend on it. A sustainable and toxin-free environment is especially important as pollution rises and global warming becomes a reality. Therefore, we need to implement practices that encourage the use of products that are less harmful to humans and the environment.

Common Household Accidents

Regardless of how careful we are, accidents happen, and they happen frequently. Common examples of household accidents include falls, tripping over objects, wounds from mishandling knives, kitchen fires, and fires caused by faulty electrical circuits. The potential for household accidents can be dramatically reduced by taking appropriate preventative measures.

Seek professional help and services if we cannot mitigate the problem ourselves. Often, this is the best option because a poor job may exacerbate the problem

Guidelines for a Healthy and Safe Home

We all deserve a healthy and happy home, but it is up to us to create such a place. Our home provides refuge from wildlife and harsh weather like flooding, earthquakes, and storms. Poor housing may offer limited protection from severe storms, which can affect our mental health and physical well-being. Your house ultimately guarantees your well-being.

Keep Your Home Tidy

Maintaining cleanliness in your home reduces the likelihood of pest invasions and exposure to harmful contaminants. Ensure your living space remains tidy by implementing strategies to prevent the entry of contaminants, establishing easy-to-clean surfaces, and minimizing clutter. Use a damp mop or cloth for cleaning tasks, and follow the instructions provided on cleaning product labels. Always keep cleaning products out of the reach of children, as tragic incidents have occurred where young children ingested dangerous chemicals, resulting in injury or death.

Keep the Home Dry

Wet surfaces support the growth of mold and fungi, enabling them to multiply quickly. Damp environments invite dust mites, cockroaches, and rodents to thrive. These pests can spread disease and dirt throughout the house. Never overlook plumbing issues; any structural leaks should be addressed immediately, including drainage problems. Delaying maintenance can cost you your well-being.

Keep Your Home Well-Ventilated

The supply of fresh air is irreplaceable. Fresh air helps reduce exposure to indoor allergy triggers and other contaminants. Use exhaust fans and open windows, especially when cleaning, cooking, or using certain chemicals, such as pesticides.

Keep Your Home Pest-Free

Every pest, from cockroaches to mice and rats, requires food, water, and shelter to survive. Maintain a pest-free environment by storing food (including pet food) in containers that pests cannot infiltrate, repairing leaks, sealing cracks in floors, walls, and ceilings, minimizing clutter, and keeping garbage stored outdoors in lidded containers. If pests have already become an issue, employ methods such as sticky traps and baits stored in enclosed containers or explore alternative non-chemical management approaches. If pesticides are necessary, adhere to recommendations for selecting, applying, storing, and disposing of them safely.

Keep Your Home Safe

Within the confines of a home, a plethora of injuries can occur, ranging from falls and burns to poisonings. Vulnerable populations, such as children and older adults, face elevated risks for specific types of injuries. To maintain safety, diligently label and store all chemicals, medicines, and personal-care products. Take precautions by securing loose rugs, eliminating sharp surfaces in children's play areas, and utilizing smoke and carbon monoxide detectors. These measures collectively contribute to the safety and well-being of all household occupants.

Maintain the Home

Homes that are not properly maintained are more likely to experience issues such as pests, moisture, deteriorating lead paint, and structural problems. Regularly inspect, clean, and repair your home. Address small repairs and problems before they escalate into larger, more expensive issues.

Keep a First-Aid Kit at Home

Having a well-stocked first-aid kit at home is essential for handling minor accidents and injuries. Store it in a cool, dry place where young children cannot reach it. Your basic first-aid kit might include:

- Plasters in various sizes
- Sterile gauze dressings
- Eye dressings
- Bandages
- Safety pins
- Gloves
- Tweezers
- Scissors
- Cleansing wipes
- Tape
- A thermometer
- Rash cream
- Insect bite relief
- Antiseptic cream
- Painkillers

- Antihistamines
- Distilled water for cleaning wounds
- Eye wash

Even the smallest particles may seem harmless, but they can cause various adverse health effects. Do not hesitate to seek help if you need it. Obtain professional services if a friend cannot resolve the problem. When it comes to your health, always be diligent—because health is the greatest wealth.

List of Numbers to Contact

The most known number for emergencies is 911. This number is used for life-threatening situations such as fires, accidental poisoning, falls, or if a person is unconscious. Another important number to have readily available is the National Capital Poison Center @ (800) 222-1222.

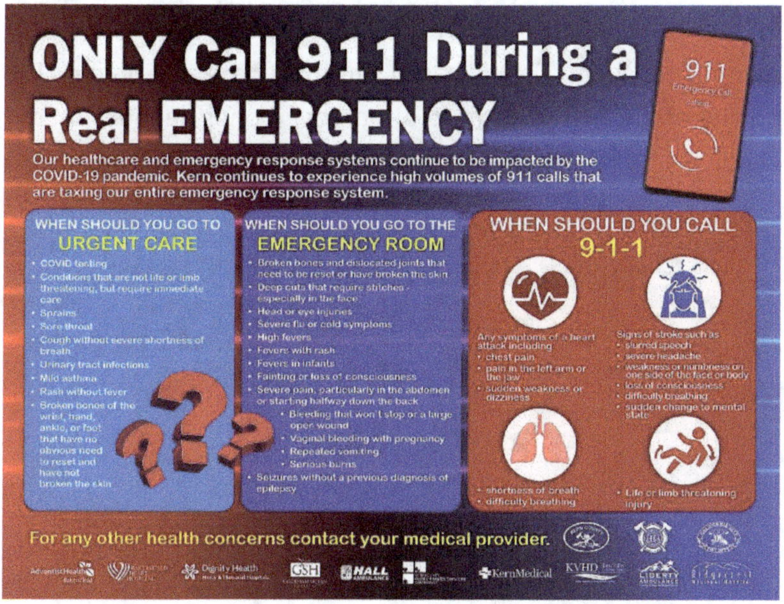

Lastly, you should create a list of important contact names and phone numbers that are easily accessible. Ensure that everyone living in the house knows where to find the emergency numbers in case of an emergency.

The list of important contact numbers should include the following:

- Local fire department
- Local hospitals
- Personal emergency contact list
- Doctor's office
- Pharmacy

It is our responsibility to maintain our homes and keep them safe and healthy. The best way to achieve this is by becoming aware of the different threats that can occur and how to prevent or mitigate them. This is based on awareness and action. The quality of our lives and those of our loved ones depends on our actions.

Emergency Contact Sheet

FOR EMERGENCY SERVICES: DIAL 911

The best time to prepare for an emergency is before it happens. Fill out this sheet and keep it near each phone. Update the sheet when necessary, and be sure to let family, babysitters, and others know that it is available.

EMERGENCY NUMBERS

Poison Control Center: **1-800-222-1222**

Hospital Name: Phone:

Doctor's Name: Phone:

Dentist's Name: Phone:

Pharmacy Name: Phone:

Health Insurance Plan:

Policy #: Phone:

FAMILY CONTACT NUMBERS

Parents' Names:

Kids' Names:

Address:

City: State: Zip:

Home Phone:

Mom Cell #: Mom Work #:

Dad Cell #: Dad Work #:

Emergency Contact 1

Name:

Relationship:

Phone:

Emergency Contact 2

Name:

Relationship:

Phone:

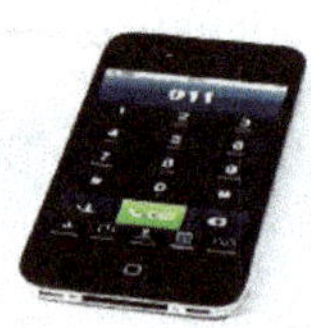

In an emergency, call 911 or your child's doctor. Before your child gets sick, speak with your doctor about the best way to handle an injury, illness, or emergency.

REFERENCES:

"Methodist Health System. (n.d.). *Your shoes may be making you sick*. Retrieved from https://bestcare.org/news/your-shoes-may-be-making-you-sick

Rhomberg, L. R., et al. (2018). A bounding quantitative cancer risk assessment for occupational exposures to asphalt emissions during road paving operations. *Critical Reviews in Toxicology, 48*(9), 713-737. https://doi.org/10.1080/10408444.2018.1528208

PT Floor Covering. (n.d.). *Why you may want to reconsider wearing shoes inside*. Retrieved from https://www.ptfloors.com/post/why-you-may-want-to-reconsider-wearing-shoes-inside#

Franklin, S., et al. (2015). Barefoot vs common footwear: A systematic review of the kinematic, kinetic, and muscle activity differences during walking. *Gait & Posture, 42*(3), 230-239. https://doi.org/10.1016/j.gaitpost.2015.05.019

Samaritan Health Services. (2021, August 11). *Going barefoot? Take smart care of your feet*. Retrieved from https://www.samhealth.org/about-samaritan/news-search/2021/08/11/be-smart-about-going-barefoot

Lambert, M. R., & Skelly, D. K. (2016). Diverse sources for endocrine disruption in the wild. *Endocrine Disruptors, 4*(1). https://doi.org/10.1080/23273747.2016.1148803

Vionic Shoes. (n.d.). *Why you shouldn't wear shoes in the house*. Retrieved from https://www.vionicshoes.com/blog/why-you-shouldnt-wear-shoes-in-the-house/

EuroScience. (n.d.). *The gross science explaining why you should take your shoes off while indoors*. Retrieved from https://www.euroscience.org/the-gross-science-explaining-why-you-should-take-your-shoes-off-while-indoors

CNN. (2023, December 7). *Why you should remove your shoes at home: Germs and wellness*. Retrieved from https://www.cnn.com/2023/12/07/health/remove-shoes-germs-wellness/index.html

Realtor.com. (n.d.). *What happens when you wear shoes in the house?*. Retrieved from https://www.realtor.com/advice/home-improvement/what-happens-when-you-wear-shoes-in-the-house/?cid=sem_7537312749_20548394769__:G:s&s_kwcid=AL!15120!3!!!!x!!&gad_source=1&gclid=EAIaIQobChMI3ITq6ZObhQMVf6VaBR33owcVEAMYASAAEgIh1PD_BwE&gclsrc=aw.ds

CiriScience. (n.d.). *Study reveals high bacteria levels on footwear*. Retrieved from https://ciriscience.org/ieq-measurement/study-reveals-high-bacteria-levels-on-footwear/

University of Houston. (n.d.). *Shoes indoors: Making an impact*. Retrieved from https://www.uh.edu/magazine/2017-fall/making-an-impact/shoes-indoors.php

Austin, G. (2022, November 30). 7 harmful side effects of plastic water bottles. *Weo*. Retrieved from https://we-o.com/blog/7-harmful-side-effects-of-plastic-water-bottles/

Borunda, A. (2019, March 18). This whale had more than 88 pounds of plastic in its stomach when it died. *National Geographic*. Retrieved from https://www.nationalgeographic.com/environment/article/whale-dies-88-pounds-plastic-philippines

U.S. Geological Survey. (n.d.). *Tap water study detects PFAS "forever chemicals" across the U.S.* Retrieved from https://www.usgs.gov/news/national-news-release/tap-water-study-detects-pfas-forever-chemicals-across-us

Office H2O. (2020, February 27). *Why are disposable water bottles harmful to the environment?* Retrieved from https://www.officeh2o.com/blog/water-news/why-are-disposable-water-bottles-harmful-to-the-environment/

Centers for Disease Control and Prevention. (2022, September 9). *Commercially bottled water*. Retrieved from https://www.cdc.gov/healthywater/drinking/bottled/index.html

Environmental Protection Agency. (2023, November 30). *Drinking water regulations*. Retrieved from https://www.epa.gov/dwreginfo/drinking-water-regulations

Environmental Protection Agency. (2024, January 25). *Basic information about lead in drinking water*. Retrieved from https://www.epa.gov/ground-water-and-drinking-water/basic-information-about-lead-drinking-water

Environmental Working Group. (n.d.). *EWG Tap Water Database*. Retrieved from https://www.ewg.org/tapwater/system.php?pws=FL4130871

Natural Resources Defense Council. (2023, September 13). *Bottled water vs. tap water*. Retrieved from https://www.nrdc.org/stories/bottled-water-vs-tap-water

Innes, R., & Cory, D. (2001). The economics of safe drinking water. *Land Economics, 77*(1), 94–117. https://doi.org/10.2307/3146983

Garcia-Bengochea, J. I. (1983). Protecting water supply aquifers in areas using deepwell wastewater disposal. *Journal (American Water Works Association), 75*(6), 288–291. http://www.jstor.org/stable/41271698

Raj, S. D. (2005). Bottled water: How safe is it? *Water Environment Research, 77*(7), 3013–3018. http://www.jstor.org/stable/25045920

The Facts About Water. (n.d.). *Setting the record straight*. Retrieved from https://thefactsaboutwater.org/press-room/correct-clarify/setting-record-straight/

CBC News. (n.d.). *Bottle vs. tap: 7 things to know about drinking water*. Retrieved from https://www.cbc.ca/news/health/bottle-vs-tap-7-things-to-know-about-drinking-water-1.2774182

International Bottled Water Association. (n.d.). *Bottled water*. Retrieved from https://bottledwater.org/types-of-water-municipal-water/

Pentair. (n.d.). *Where does bottled water come from?* Retrieved from https://www.pentair.com/en-us/water-softening-filtration/blog/where-does-bottled-water-come-from.html

Consumer Reports. (n.d.). *Arsenic in some bottled water brands at unsafe levels*. Retrieved from https://www.consumerreports.org/water-quality/arsenic-in-some-bottled-water-brands-at-unsafe-levels-a1198655241/

Agency for Toxic Substances and Disease Registry. (1995). *Health consultation for Metaltec Aerosystems, Franklin Borough, Sussex County, NJ* (CERCLIS No. NJD002517472).

Agency for Toxic Substances and Disease Registry. (1994). *Site review and update for Brick Township Landfill, Brick Township, Ocean County, NJ* (CERCLIS No. NJD980505176).

Agency for Toxic Substances and Disease Registry. (1992). *Health assessment for A.O. Polymer, Sparta Township, Sussex County, NJ* (CERCLIS No. NJD030253355).

Environmental Law Centre. (n.d.). *Toxic household products*. Retrieved from http://www.elc.org.uk/pages/envirohome.htm

Wouters, I. M., Douwes, J., Doekes, G., Thorne, P. S., Brunekreef, B., & Heederik, D. J. J. (2000). Increased levels of markers of microbial exposure in homes with indoor storage of organic household waste. *Applied and Environmental Microbiology, 66*(2), 627-631. Retrieved from http://aem.asm.org/cgi/content/abstract/66/2/627

Air Purifiers and Filters. (n.d.). *Contaminants*. Retrieved from http://www.airpurifiersandfilters.com/contaminants.php

Canada Mortgage and Housing Corporation. (n.d.). *Indoor air quality and health*. Retrieved from http://www.cmhc-schl.gc.ca/en/co/maho/yohoyohe/inaiqu/inaiqu_006.cfm

USA Water Quality. (n.d.). *Health*. Retrieved from http://www.usawaterquality.org/themes/health/

U.S. Environmental Protection Agency. (n.d.). *Contaminants*. Retrieved from http://www.epa.gov/safewater/contaminants/index.html

Brent, R. (2009). *Pregnancy and radiation exposure*. Health Physics Society. Retrieved from http://www.hps.org/hpspublications/articles/pregnancyandradiationexposureinfosheet.html

Knave, B. (n.d.). Electric and magnetic fields and health outcomes. *Journal of Environmental Health, 49*(1), 1-31. Retrieved from http://www.eagosh.org/eagosh-files/articles_presentations_infos/radiation/annex_ilo_electromagnetic_radiation_health_aspects.pdf

Massachusetts Children's Health Coalition. (n.d.). *Home and garage safety*. Retrieved from http://www.mchc.org/ipc/poisoninghazards/HomeandGarageSafety.pdf

Society for the Prevention of Cruelty to Animals International. (n.d.). *What poisons lurk in your home and yard?* Retrieved from http://www.spcai.org/learn/animal-care-advice/item/125-what-poisons-lurk-in-your-home-and-yard?.html

UConn Health Poison Control. (n.d.). *Poisons index*. Retrieved from http://poisoncontrol.uchc.edu/poisons/index.htm

Kuehn, C. M., Mueller, B. A., Checkoway, H., & Williams, M. (2007). Risk of malformations associated with residential proximity to hazardous waste sites in Washington State. *Environmental Research, 103*(3), 405-412. https://doi.org/10.1016/j.envres.2007.01.007

World Health Organization. (2007, June). *Electromagnetic fields and public health: Fact sheet No. 322*. Retrieved from http://www.who.int/mediacentre/factsheets/fs322/en/index.html. Retrieved January 23, 2008.

American Medical Association. (1994, December). *Report 7 of the Council on Scientific Affairs (I-94)*. Retrieved from http://www.ama-assn.org/ama/no-index/about-ama/13682.shtml. Retrieved December 3, 2009.

Feychting, M., Jonsson, F., Pedersen, N. L., & Ahlbom, A. (2003). Occupational magnetic field exposure and neurodegenerative disease. *Epidemiology, 14*(4), 413-419. https://doi.org/10.1097/01.EDE.0000071409.23291.7b

Mother Nature Network. (n.d.). *How lawn chemicals and herbicides affect dogs*. Retrieved from http://www.mnn.com/family/pets/stories/how-lawn-chemicals-and-herbicides-affect-dogs

Ahlbom A (2001). "Neurodegenerative diseases, suicide and depressive symptoms in relation to EMF". *Bioelectromagnetics* **Suppl 5**: S132–43. doi:10.1002/1521-186X(2001)22:5+<::AID-BEM1029>3.0.CO;2-V. PMID 11170123.

Better Health Victoria. (n.d.). *Indoor air quality*. Retrieved from http://www.betterhealth.vic.gov.au/BHCV2...

U.S. Environmental Protection Agency. (n.d.). *Mold*. Retrieved from http://www.epa.gov/mold/index.html

Chem-Tox. (n.d.). *Pesticides*. Retrieved from http://www.chem-tox.com/pesticides/

Radon.com. (n.d.). *Radon information*. Retrieved from http://www.radon.com/radon/radon_EPA.html

U.S. Environmental Protection Agency. (n.d.). *Radon: Where you live*. Retrieved from http://www.epa.gov/radon/whereyoulive.html

Home Air Purifier Expert. (n.d.). *Radon*. Retrieved from http://www.home-air-purifier-expert.com/radon.html

U.S. Environmental Protection Agency. (n.d.). *Radon in water*. Retrieved from http://www.epa.gov/radon/rnwater.html

Environmental Law Centre. (n.d.). *Environmental home*. Retrieved from http://www.elc.org.uk/pages/envirohome.htm

Wouters, I. M., Douwes, J., Doekes, G., Thorne, P. S., Brunekreef, B., & Heederik, D. J. J. (2000). Increased levels of markers of microbial exposure in homes with indoor storage of organic household waste. *Applied and Environmental Microbiology, 66*(2), 627-631. https://doi.org/10.1128/AEM.66.2.627-631.2000

N/A. (n.d.). *Abstract: Electric and magnetic fields and health outcomes*. *Applied and Environmental Microbiology, 66*(2), 627. Retrieved from http://aem.asm.org/cgi/content/abstract/66/2/627

Air Purifiers and Filters. (n.d.). *Contaminants*. Retrieved from http://www.airpurifiersandfilters.com/contaminants.php

Canada Mortgage and Housing Corporation. (n.d.). *Indoor air quality and health*. Retrieved from http://www.cmhc-schl.gc.ca/en/co/maho/yohoyohe/inaiqu/inaiqu_006.cfm

USA Water Quality. (n.d.). *Health*. Retrieved from http://www.usawaterquality.org/themes/health/

U.S. Environmental Protection Agency. (n.d.). *Contaminants*. Retrieved from http://www.epa.gov/safewater/contaminants/index.html

Brent, R. (2009). *Pregnancy and radiation exposure*. Health Physics Society. Retrieved from http://www.hps.org/hpspublications/articles/pregnancyandradiationexposureinfosheet.html

Health Physics Society. (n.d.). *Pregnancy and radiation exposure*. Retrieved from http://www.hps.org/hpspublications/articles/pregnancyandradiationexposureinfosheet.html

Knave, B. (n.d.). Electric and magnetic fields and health outcomes. *Journal of Environmental Health, 49*(1), 1-31.

International Labour Organization. (n.d.). *Electromagnetic radiation: Health aspects*. Retrieved from http://www.eagosh.org/eagosh-files/articles_presentations_infos/radiation/annex_ilo_electromagnetic_radiation_health_aspects.pdf

Massachusetts Children's Health Coalition. (n.d.). *Home and garage safety*. Retrieved from http://www.mchc.org/ipc/poisoninghazards/HomeandGarageSafety.pdf

Society for the Prevention of Cruelty to Animals International. (n.d.). *What poisons lurk in your home and yard?* Retrieved from http://www.spcai.org/learn/animal-care-advice/item/125-what-poisons-lurk-in-your-home-and-yard?.html

UConn Health Poison Control. (n.d.). *Poisons index*. Retrieved from http://poisoncontrol.uchc.edu/poisons/index.htm

American Psychiatric Association. (2023, April 12). *Air pollution's impact on mental health*. https://www.psychiatry.org/news-room/apa-blogs/air-pollutions-impact-on-mental-health#:~:text=The%20lead%20author%20of%20the,those%20who%20breathe%20cleaner%20air.%E2%80%9D

Note: *For entries where no specific publication date is provided, "n.d." (no date) is used.*

GLOSSARY

- **Accidents**: Unplanned events that can result in injury or damage.
- **Acetone**: A volatile, flammable liquid used as a solvent, commonly found in nail polish remover and other cleaning products.
- **Acute exposure**: Short-term exposure to a harmful substance that can cause immediate adverse effects.
- **Aerosol sprays**: Products that dispense a substance in a fine mist, which can include air fresheners, paints, and cleaning agents.
- **Air fresheners**: Products designed to mask or eliminate unpleasant odors in indoor environments.
- **Allergens**: Substances that can trigger allergic reactions, such as pollen, dust mites, or pet dander.
- **Allergies**: Overreactions of the immune system to normally harmless substances, resulting in symptoms like sneezing, itching, or swelling.
- **Alzheimer's disease**: A progressive neurological disorder that causes memory loss, confusion, and other cognitive impairments.
- **Ammonia**: A pungent gas used in cleaning products and fertilizers, known to cause respiratory and eye irritation.
- **Anti-slip strips**: Adhesive strips applied to surfaces to prevent slipping and reduce the risk of falls.
- **Asbestos**: A group of naturally occurring fibrous minerals that are hazardous when inhaled, leading to serious respiratory diseases.

- **Asphyxiation**: A condition caused by a lack of oxygen, which can lead to suffocation or choking.
- **Asthma**: A chronic respiratory condition characterized by inflammation and narrowing of the airways, leading to breathing difficulties.
- **Autoimmune diseases**: Conditions where the immune system mistakenly attacks the body's own tissues.
- **Backyards**: Outdoor areas adjacent to a house, often used for recreation, gardening, or relaxation.
- **Bacteria**: Microscopic single-celled organisms that can be beneficial or harmful, depending on the type and context.
- **Bathtubs**: Fixtures used for bathing, which can pose risks of slips and falls if not properly maintained.
- **Benzene**: A toxic, flammable liquid used in industrial processes and found in some household products, linked to health risks such as cancer.
- **Biohazard signs**: Warnings indicating the presence of biological materials that pose a risk to health, such as pathogens or toxic substances.
- **Biological pollutants**: Contaminants of biological origin, including mold, bacteria, and viruses, that can affect health.
- **Bite fever**: A condition caused by bites from insects or animals, leading to symptoms like fever and rash.
- **Bleach**: A strong disinfectant and whitening agent commonly used in cleaning and laundry, which can irritate the skin and respiratory tract.

- **Brain cancer**: A malignant tumor that develops in the brain tissue, affecting cognitive functions and potentially leading to serious health issues.
- **Brown-banded cockroaches**: A type of cockroach known for its brown bands across its body, which can be carriers of allergens and pathogens.
- **Brucellosis**: An infectious disease caused by bacteria of the genus *Brucella*, often contracted through unpasteurized dairy products or contact with infected animals.
- **Bubonic plague**: A serious infectious disease caused by the bacterium *Yersinia pestis*, transmitted by fleas and characterized by swollen lymph nodes (buboes).
- **Burning sensations**: A discomfort or pain often associated with chemical exposure, burns, or certain medical conditions.
- **Burns**: Injuries caused by heat, chemicals, or electricity, leading to damage of the skin and potentially deeper tissues.
- **Butanal**: A volatile organic compound used in industrial applications and found in some cleaning products.
- **Butylbenzene**: A chemical compound used in industrial processes, known for its potential health hazards including respiratory irritation.
- **Cancer**: A group of diseases characterized by uncontrolled cell growth that can spread to other parts of the body, with various types including skin, lung, and breast cancer.

- **Carbon monoxide (CO)**: A colorless, odorless gas produced by incomplete combustion of carbon-containing fuels, which can be harmful or fatal when inhaled in high concentrations.
- **Carcinogens**: Substances or agents that can cause cancer, either by directly damaging DNA or by causing other cellular changes.
- **Cardiovascular system**: The system comprising the heart and blood vessels responsible for circulating blood throughout the body, which can be affected by various environmental and lifestyle factors.
- **Chagas disease**: A tropical disease caused by the parasite *Trypanosoma cruzi*, transmitted by triatomine bugs and potentially leading to heart and digestive issues.
- **Chemical exposure**: Contact with chemicals that can be harmful, either through inhalation, ingestion, or skin contact, potentially leading to health problems.
- **Child-proofed**: Measures taken to make an environment safer for children by removing or securing potential hazards.
- **Child-proofing**: The process of making a space safe for children by addressing potential dangers such as sharp objects, choking hazards, and unsafe furniture.
- **Children's play areas**: Designated spaces for children to play, which should be designed with safety features to prevent injuries.
- **Chlorofluorocarbons (CFCs)**: Chemical compounds used in refrigeration and air conditioning, which can damage the ozone layer and contribute to global warming.

- **Cholera**: A bacterial infection of the small intestine caused by *Vibrio cholerae*, leading to severe diarrhea and dehydration.
- **Chromosomal mutations**: Changes in the structure or number of chromosomes that can lead to genetic disorders or increase the risk of diseases.
- **Chronic disease**: A long-lasting health condition that can be controlled but not cured, such as diabetes, heart disease, or arthritis.
- **Chronic exposure**: Continuous or repeated exposure to a harmful substance over a long period, potentially leading to adverse health effects.
- **Chronic obstructive pulmonary disease (COPD)**: A group of lung diseases, including emphysema and chronic bronchitis, that cause breathing difficulties and reduced airflow.
- **Cigarettes**: Tobacco products rolled in paper for smoking, which contain harmful chemicals that can lead to various health problems, including cancer and respiratory diseases.
- **Cleaning**: The process of removing dirt, dust, and other impurities from surfaces, which is essential for maintaining a healthy and safe environment.
- **Clutter**: An accumulation of items that are disorganized or unnecessary, which can pose tripping hazards and affect mental well-being.
- **Cockroaches**: Common household pests known for spreading diseases, allergens, and triggering asthma and allergy symptoms.

- **Cognitive function**: The mental processes involved in gaining knowledge and understanding, including memory, attention, and decision-making.
- **Cognitive impairments**: Difficulties or deficits in cognitive functions, which can result from injury, disease, or environmental factors.
- **Congestion**: A condition characterized by a blocked or stuffy nose, often due to allergies, infections, or exposure to irritants.
- **Contaminants**: Substances that pollute or make a substance impure, which can be biological, chemical, or physical in nature.
- **Corrosive substances**: Chemicals that can cause damage to skin, eyes, or other materials upon contact, such as acids and alkalis.
- **Cortisol**: A stress hormone produced by the adrenal glands, which regulates various bodily functions and responses to stress.
- **Cracks**: Openings or splits in surfaces that can allow pests, moisture, and contaminants to enter or cause structural weaknesses.
- **Craft materials**: Supplies used in creative activities that can sometimes contain hazardous chemicals or small parts posing choking hazards.
- **Crawling infants**: Babies in the developmental stage of crawling, who are vulnerable to potential hazards like small objects or toxins on the floor.

- **Cuts**: Injuries caused by sharp objects that break the skin, which can range from minor scratches to severe lacerations.
- **Dampness**: The presence of moisture in the air or on surfaces, which can promote mold growth and create an unhealthy indoor environment.
- **Debris**: Scattered fragments of waste or remains that can pose safety hazards in various settings.
- **Decluttering**: The process of removing unnecessary or unwanted items from a space to create a safer and more organized environment.
- **Dementia**: A group of symptoms affecting memory, thinking, and social abilities, which interfere with daily life and are typically caused by brain diseases.
- **Depression**: A mental health disorder characterized by persistent feelings of sadness, loss of interest, and other emotional and physical symptoms.
- **Deserts**: Arid regions with little precipitation, which can pose environmental and survival challenges due to extreme conditions.
- **Dioxin**: A toxic chemical compound found in the environment, primarily as a byproduct of industrial processes, which can cause serious health issues.
- **Discoloration**: Changes in the natural color of a material or surface, often indicating damage or contamination.
- **Dizziness**: A sensation of spinning or loss of balance, which can result from various causes such as dehydration, medication, or health conditions.

- **Drain cleaners**: Chemical substances designed to clear clogs in drains, which can be highly corrosive and dangerous if improperly handled.
- **Dried rat urine**: Residue from rodent infestations, which can carry harmful pathogens and pose health risks.
- **Dry-cleaned clothing**: Garments cleaned using solvents instead of water, which may retain chemical residues that can irritate sensitive individuals.
- **Dust**: Fine particles of matter that accumulate in the environment and can contain allergens, bacteria, and other harmful substances.
- **Dysentery**: An intestinal infection that causes severe diarrhea, often caused by bacteria, viruses, or parasites.
- **Earthquakes**: Natural disasters caused by the sudden release of energy in the Earth's crust, resulting in ground shaking and potential destruction.
- **Eastern equine**: A viral infection, specifically Eastern equine encephalitis (EEE), transmitted by mosquitoes and affecting the brain.
- **Emergency numbers**: Contact numbers for essential services like fire, police, and medical emergencies, crucial for immediate response.
- **Emergency supplies**: Items kept on hand to address emergencies, such as first aid kits, food, water, and other essentials.
- **EMF (Electromagnetic Fields)**: Invisible areas of energy produced by electricity flow, which can affect health under prolonged or high exposure.

- **Emotional attachment**: A strong, often sentimental connection to objects or people, which can impact decisions about keeping or discarding items.
- **Encephalitis**: Inflammation of the brain caused by infections, autoimmune reactions, or other factors, potentially leading to serious neurological symptoms.
- **Engineered wood fiber**: A type of material used in playgrounds and landscaping that provides a safe, cushioned surface.
- **Environment**: The surrounding conditions, including air, water, and land, that affect living organisms and overall quality of life.
- **Environmental awareness**: The understanding and concern about environmental issues and the impact of human activities on the planet.
- **Excessive sneezing**: Frequent, intense sneezing that can be caused by allergens, infections, or irritants in the environment.
- **Explosives**: Substances that can cause explosions and pose significant safety risks if mishandled or improperly stored.
- **Extreme panic**: An intense fear or anxiety response that can lead to irrational behavior and difficulty in managing emergencies.
- **Falls**: Accidental drops to the ground or lower levels, which can result in injuries, especially in vulnerable populations like children and the elderly.
- **Fatigue**: A state of physical or mental exhaustion that can result from stress, illness, or environmental factors.

- **Feces**: Waste material excreted from the digestive tract through the anus, which can contain pathogens and pose health risks if not properly managed.
- **Fences**: Barriers used to enclose areas for safety, privacy, or security purposes, often around properties, gardens, or children's play areas.
- **Fertilizers**: Substances applied to soil or plants to provide essential nutrients, which can pose environmental risks if not used responsibly.
- **Fire safety plan**: A comprehensive strategy designed to prevent fire incidents and provide instructions on how to respond in case of a fire.
- **First-aid kit**: A collection of supplies and equipment used to provide initial medical treatment in case of an injury or emergency.
- **Flammable liquids**: Liquids that can easily catch fire, such as gasoline, alcohol, and certain cleaning agents, requiring careful storage and handling.
- **Fleas**: Small, wingless insects that feed on the blood of mammals and birds, often spreading diseases and causing allergic reactions.
- **Flooding**: Overflow of water onto normally dry land, which can cause property damage, displacement, and health hazards.
- **Formaldehyde**: A colorless, strong-smelling gas used in building materials and household products, which can cause respiratory problems and is considered a carcinogen.

- **Forum of International Societies Environmental Committee**: A committee focused on addressing environmental issues and promoting sustainable practices on a global scale.
- **Fungi**: A group of spore-producing organisms, including molds and yeasts, that can cause health problems and damage to property.
- **Fungicides**: Chemical substances used to kill or inhibit the growth of fungi, often used in agriculture and gardening.
- **Fungus**: A type of organism, such as mold or mildew, that grows in damp environments and can cause structural damage and health issues.
- **Furan**: A toxic compound found in some industrial processes and as a byproduct of food processing, which can pose health risks.
- **Furnishings**: Furniture and other decorative items in a home or office that contribute to interior aesthetics and comfort.
- **Furniture polish**: A product used to clean and protect wood surfaces, which may contain chemicals that can be harmful if ingested or inhaled.
- **Gases**: Airborne substances that can be hazardous if inhaled, such as carbon monoxide or radon, which can accumulate indoors and affect air quality.
- **Gastroenteritis**: An inflammation of the stomach and intestines, typically resulting in diarrhea, vomiting, and abdominal pain, often caused by bacterial or viral infections.

- **Genetic damage**: Harm to DNA that can result in mutations and contribute to the development of diseases like cancer.
- **German cockroach**: A small species of cockroach known for infesting homes and spreading allergens and pathogens.
- **Glues and adhesives**: Substances used to bond materials together, which can release toxic fumes and pose choking hazards if ingested.
- **Grassy areas**: Open spaces covered with grass, often used for recreational activities and landscaping, but may need maintenance to prevent pests.
- **Habituation**: A psychological process where repeated exposure to a stimulus reduces an individual's response to it, often seen in hoarding behavior.
- **Handrail stability**: The security and sturdiness of handrails, crucial for preventing falls and accidents, especially on stairways.
- **Hantavirus**: A virus transmitted by rodents, especially through contact with their urine, feces, or saliva, which can cause severe respiratory illnesses.
- **Harmful substances**: Chemicals or materials that can cause harm to health or the environment when ingested, inhaled, or contacted.
- **Hazardous**: Describes substances or situations that pose a risk of causing harm or danger, requiring caution and safety measures.
- **Hazards**: Potential sources of harm or danger, including physical, chemical, biological, and ergonomic risks.

- **Headaches**: Pain in the head or upper neck region, which can result from various causes such as tension, allergies, or exposure to certain chemicals.
- **Health**: The overall condition of a person's body and mind, including physical, mental, and social well-being, free from illness or injury.
- **Health risks**: Factors or conditions that increase the likelihood of developing health problems or diseases.
- **Heart attacks**: Medical emergencies caused by blocked blood flow to the heart, which can result in severe chest pain and require immediate attention.
- **Hemorrhagic fever**: A group of illnesses caused by viruses, characterized by fever and bleeding disorders, often transmitted by insects or rodents.
- **Herbicides**: Chemicals used to kill unwanted plants or weeds, which can pose health risks if misused or overexposed.
- **High-frequency EMFs (Electromagnetic Fields)**: Electromagnetic waves at high frequencies, often emitted by electronic devices, which can affect human health under certain conditions.
- **High-power electric lines**: Electrical transmission lines that carry high voltage, posing potential health risks such as electromagnetic radiation exposure.
- **Hoarding**: A psychological condition characterized by excessive accumulation of items and an inability to discard them, leading to cluttered and unsafe living conditions.

- **Home fixtures**: Permanent installations in a home, such as lighting, plumbing, and cabinetry, which need regular maintenance for safety and functionality.
- **Hormone**: Chemical messengers in the body that regulate various physiological processes, including growth, metabolism, and mood.
- **Household accidents**: Unintended incidents that occur in the home, often resulting in injuries such as falls, burns, and cuts.
- **Household appliances**: Electrical or mechanical devices used in the home for various tasks, which require proper use and maintenance to prevent accidents.
- **Hygiene**: Practices and conditions that help maintain health and prevent the spread of diseases, such as regular cleaning and handwashing.
- **Inadequate nutrition**: A condition where a diet lacks essential nutrients, leading to health problems like weakened immunity and impaired growth.
- **Indoor air pollutants**: Contaminants found in indoor air, including dust, mold, smoke, and chemicals, which can affect respiratory health and overall well-being.
- **Indoor air pollution**: Contamination of the indoor environment by various pollutants such as smoke, chemicals, mold, and allergens that can negatively affect human health.
- **Indoor air quality**: The quality of the air inside buildings and structures, affected by factors like ventilation, humidity, and the presence of pollutants.

- **Indoor pollutants**: Substances or particles in the air inside buildings that can cause harm to health, including dust, mold, volatile organic compounds (VOCs), and chemicals.
- **Infestation**: The presence of large numbers of pests, such as insects or rodents, in a space, which can lead to contamination and health hazards.
- **Infestations**: Multiple occurrences or situations where pests invade spaces, causing potential health and structural issues.
- **Injuries**: Physical harm or damage to a body resulting from accidents, falls, or other harmful incidents.
- **Injury-involved accidents**: Accidents that result in physical harm or bodily injuries, often requiring medical attention.
- **Injury-related deaths**: Fatalities resulting from accidents or injuries, emphasizing the need for safety precautions.
- **Insecticides**: Chemical substances used to kill or control insects, often applied in agricultural, residential, and commercial settings.
- **Insects**: Small, six-legged arthropods that can become pests, causing damage to crops, property, and health.
- **Laptops**: Portable personal computers used for various tasks, which can emit electromagnetic fields (EMFs) and generate heat.
- **Lead**: A toxic metal found in old paints, pipes, and other materials, which can cause serious health issues like neurological damage when ingested or inhaled.

- **LED light bulbs**: Energy-efficient lighting options that use light-emitting diodes (LEDs) and are safer and more sustainable than traditional incandescent bulbs.
- **Leprosy**: A chronic infectious disease caused by *Mycobacterium leprae*, affecting the skin, nerves, and mucous membranes.
- **Leptospira**: A genus of bacteria that can cause leptospirosis, a zoonotic disease transmitted through contact with contaminated water or animal urine.
- **Leptospirosis**: A bacterial infection that affects humans and animals, often contracted through contact with water contaminated by animal urine.
- **Lymphocytic choriomeningitis (LCMV)**: A viral infection transmitted by rodents, which can cause meningitis or encephalitis in humans.
- **Malaria**: A life-threatening disease caused by *Plasmodium* parasites, transmitted to humans through the bites of infected mosquitoes.
- **Mammalian blood**: Blood from mammals, often discussed in the context of blood-feeding insects like fleas and mosquitoes.
- **Manufacturing**: The process of producing goods on a large scale using machinery, which can pose environmental and occupational safety risks.
- **Mental health**: A state of well-being that involves emotional, psychological, and social stability, crucial for overall quality of life.

- **Mental well-being**: The state of being comfortable, healthy, and happy, often influenced by environmental, social, and psychological factors.
- **Mess**: A state of disorder or untidiness, often requiring decluttering and cleaning to maintain a safe and healthy environment.
- **Methane**: A potent greenhouse gas and a flammable gas found in natural gas and emitted by landfills, livestock, and certain industrial activities.
- **Methylene chloride**: A volatile organic compound (VOC) used in paint removers and degreasers, which can pose significant health risks upon inhalation or exposure.
- **Mice**: Small rodents that can infest homes, spread diseases, and cause damage by gnawing on wires and structures.
- **Microbes**: Microscopic organisms, including bacteria, viruses, fungi, and protozoa, that can cause diseases or be beneficial for various applications.
- **Microwaves**: Electromagnetic waves commonly used in kitchen appliances for cooking and in communication devices, which can emit low levels of radiation.
- **Mildew**: A type of fungus that grows on damp surfaces, often causing discoloration and health issues such as respiratory problems.
- **Mites**: Tiny arthropods that can infest homes and cause allergic reactions, often found in dust, bedding, and upholstered furniture.
- **Mold**: A type of fungus that grows in damp or humid conditions, which can cause structural damage and

health issues, including respiratory problems and allergic reactions.

- **Mosquitoes**: Blood-feeding insects that can transmit diseases such as malaria, dengue, and Zika virus through their bites.
- **Moth repellents**: Substances used to deter moths from infesting clothes and fabrics, often containing chemicals like naphthalene.
- **MRI machines**: Medical imaging devices that use magnetic fields and radio waves to produce detailed images of organs and tissues, commonly used in hospitals and clinics.
- **Muscle aches**: Soreness or discomfort in the muscles, which can result from physical exertion, stress, or exposure to certain toxins.
- **Nail polish remover**: A solvent, often containing acetone or ethyl acetate, used to remove nail polish, which can be flammable and emit strong fumes.
- **Naphthalene**: A chemical compound used in mothballs and some air fresheners, which can pose health risks if inhaled or ingested.
- **Nervous system**: The network of nerve cells and fibers that transmits signals between different parts of the body, responsible for coordinating bodily functions.
- **Neurological conditions**: Disorders that affect the brain, spinal cord, and nerves, impacting movement, cognition, and sensation.

- **Nocturnal animals**: Animals that are active primarily at night, such as rodents and certain insects, which may enter homes seeking food or shelter.
- **Not-for-profit institutions**: Organizations that operate for charitable, educational, or social purposes rather than for profit, such as non-governmental organizations (NGOs) and charities.
- **NSC (National Safety Council)**: A U.S. nonprofit organization focused on promoting health and safety practices to prevent accidents and injuries.
- **Nuclear power plants**: Facilities that generate electricity through nuclear reactions, particularly nuclear fission, which involves the splitting of atomic nuclei. They pose risks such as radiation exposure and nuclear accidents.
- **Organisms**: Living entities, including bacteria, viruses, fungi, and other microscopic life forms, that can have both beneficial and harmful effects on health and the environment.
- **Outdoor pollution**: Contamination of the outdoor environment by pollutants such as vehicle emissions, industrial discharges, and particulate matter, which can harm human health and the ecosystem.
- **Oven cleaners**: Chemical products used to clean ovens, often containing strong caustic agents like sodium hydroxide that can cause burns and respiratory issues.
- **Oxidizing substances**: Chemicals that can release oxygen and cause or enhance the combustion of other materials, potentially leading to fires or explosions.

- **Packaged spray products**: Aerosol products like deodorants, cleaners, and insecticides that release fine particles or chemicals into the air, potentially causing respiratory issues and environmental pollution.
- **Paint and paint thinners**: Substances used to apply or remove paint; often contain volatile organic compounds (VOCs) that can be harmful when inhaled and contribute to indoor air pollution.
- **Paint removers**: Chemicals used to strip paint from surfaces, typically containing solvents like methylene chloride, which can be toxic if inhaled or absorbed through the skin.
- **Particulate matter**: Tiny particles suspended in the air, such as dust, soot, and smoke, which can penetrate the respiratory system and cause health issues like asthma and cardiovascular problems.
- **Pathogenic**: Referring to microorganisms, such as bacteria, viruses, or fungi, that can cause diseases or infections in humans, animals, or plants.
- **Peace lilies**: Popular indoor plants known for their air-purifying qualities, as they can remove toxins like formaldehyde and benzene from the air.
- **Peppermint oil**: An essential oil derived from the peppermint plant, often used as a natural insect repellent or for its soothing and aromatic properties.
- **Permanent markers**: Writing tools that contain ink formulated with solvents like xylene and toluene, which can release fumes harmful to inhale over prolonged periods.

- **Pesticide exposure**: Contact with chemicals used to kill pests, which can occur through inhalation, ingestion, or skin absorption and potentially lead to health issues like poisoning or cancer.
- **Pesticides**: Chemicals used to control, repel, or kill pests such as insects, weeds, and fungi, which can pose environmental and health risks when improperly handled.
- **Pests**: Unwanted organisms such as insects, rodents, or weeds that can cause harm to humans, crops, or property, often controlled through pesticides or other methods.
- **Petrochemical**: Chemical products derived from petroleum or natural gas, often used in the manufacture of plastics, fertilizers, and other materials.
- **Phthalates**: Chemical compounds used as plasticizers in various consumer products like toys, flooring, and personal care products, which can disrupt hormones and pose health risks.
- **Plastic leach phthalates**: Phthalates that leach from plastic materials into the environment or food, potentially causing hormonal disruptions and other health concerns.
- **Poisoning**: The harmful effect of ingesting, inhaling, or coming into contact with toxic substances, which can result in illness or death.
- **Pollen**: Fine powder produced by plants for fertilization, which can cause allergic reactions like hay fever and asthma in sensitive individuals.

- **Pollution**: The introduction of harmful substances or products into the environment, which can cause health problems and degrade natural resources.
- **Poor focus**: A lack of concentration or attention, which can result from environmental factors like poor indoor air quality or exposure to pollutants.
- **Poor sanitation**: Inadequate cleanliness and hygiene practices that can lead to the spread of diseases and contamination of water and food sources.
- **Poverty**: The state of having insufficient financial resources, which can limit access to basic needs, healthcare, and safe living conditions, impacting overall well-being.
- **Prickling**: A tingling or stinging sensation on the skin, often resulting from exposure to certain chemicals, allergens, or environmental conditions.
- **Proper ventilation**: The process of circulating fresh air into indoor spaces to reduce the concentration of pollutants, humidity, and odors, improving air quality.
- **Protrusions**: Parts that extend outward from a surface, potentially posing tripping, bruising, or other safety hazards.
- **Psychological distress**: A state of emotional suffering characterized by symptoms like anxiety, depression, or stress, often resulting from environmental, social, or personal factors.
- **Pulmonary syndrome**: A group of lung diseases caused by inhaling harmful substances like chemicals, dust, or biological agents, leading to respiratory distress.

- **Pulverized rubber**: Crushed or ground rubber materials often used in playground surfacing, which can contain chemicals that may pose health risks.
- **PVC flooring**: Flooring made from polyvinyl chloride (PVC), a synthetic plastic polymer that can release harmful chemicals like phthalates and VOCs over time.
- **Radar**: A system that uses radio waves to detect objects' positions, speed, and direction, commonly used in aviation, weather forecasting, and defense.
- **Radiation**: Energy emitted in the form of particles or electromagnetic waves, which can be ionizing (e.g., X-rays) or non-ionizing (e.g., microwaves) and may pose health risks.
- **Radio**: A communication device that uses radio waves to transmit and receive signals, which can also emit low levels of non-ionizing radiation.
- **Radioactive gases**: Gases that emit radiation, such as radon, which can accumulate in buildings and pose serious health risks like lung cancer.
- **Radioactive substances**: Materials that emit radiation as they decay, such as uranium, radium, and radon, which can pose health hazards through exposure.
- **Radon**: A colorless, odorless, radioactive gas formed from the natural decay of uranium in soil, which can accumulate in homes and increase lung cancer risk.
- **Radon-226**: A radioactive isotope of radon, part of the uranium-238 decay chain, which poses significant health risks due to its high radiation levels.

- **Rashes**: Red, inflamed skin caused by allergens, irritants, infections, or underlying health conditions, which can be itchy, painful, or unsightly.
- **Rats**: Rodents known for spreading diseases, contaminating food, and causing property damage by gnawing and burrowing.
- **Reactive substances**: Chemicals that readily undergo chemical changes, potentially causing explosions, fires, or toxic gas releases.
- **Recreation**: Activities done for enjoyment, relaxation, or exercise, which can contribute to physical and mental well-being.
- **Refrigerators**: Appliances used to keep food and drinks cold, which can pose safety risks such as electrical hazards or refrigerant leaks.
- **Respiratory infections**: Infections of the respiratory tract caused by bacteria, viruses, or fungi, leading to conditions like bronchitis, pneumonia, and the common cold.
- **Responsible environmental habits**: Practices that promote sustainability, reduce pollution, and protect natural resources, such as recycling and energy conservation.
- **Rocks**: Solid mineral material forming part of the earth's crust, which can contain natural sources of radiation like uranium and radium.
- **Rodents**: Small mammals like rats, mice, and squirrels that can cause property damage, spread diseases, and contaminate food supplies.

- **Roof rats**: A species of rat known for nesting in higher areas like attics and roofs, posing health and structural risks.
- **Runny nose**: A condition where excess mucus is produced in the nasal passages, often due to allergies, infections, or irritants.
- **Safe surfacing**: Materials like rubber or foam used in playgrounds and other areas to cushion falls and prevent injuries.
- **Safety**: The condition of being protected from harm or danger, which includes practices, devices, and regulations to prevent accidents and injuries.
- **Safety rules**: Guidelines or regulations designed to prevent accidents and ensure the safe operation of equipment, facilities, or activities.
- **Salivation**: The production and secretion of saliva, which can be stimulated by eating, smelling food, or as a response to certain stimuli or conditions.
- **Salmonellosis**: An infection caused by Salmonella bacteria, often resulting from consuming contaminated food or water. Symptoms include diarrhea, fever, and abdominal cramps.
- **Sand**: A granular material composed of finely divided rock and mineral particles. It is commonly used in construction, landscaping, and as a natural filtration system.
- **Satellite Stations**: Facilities used for broadcasting or receiving television, radio, or internet signals. These

stations work as intermediate relay points to ensure signal transmission over long distances.

- **Scalding**: A type of burn caused by hot liquids or steam. Scald injuries are common in households, especially involving hot water or cooking oil.
- **Seasonal Affective Disorder**: A type of depression that occurs at a specific time of year, usually in the winter when daylight hours are shorter. It is treated with light therapy, medication, or psychotherapy.
- **Self-Closing Gates**: Gates designed to close automatically after being opened, commonly used in swimming pool areas or child-proofing homes to prevent accidents.
- **Sharp Edges**: Points or borders on objects that can cause cuts or injuries. These are often found in furniture, tools, or household items.
- **Silent Killer**: A term used to describe hazards like carbon monoxide, which are deadly but difficult to detect without specific detectors.
- **Skin Irritation**: Inflammation or discomfort on the skin caused by contact with irritants, allergens, or prolonged exposure to moisture.
- **Skin Symptoms**: Observable signs on the skin, such as redness, itching, or rashes, indicating various health conditions or reactions.
- **Sleep Disturbances**: Problems with sleeping, such as insomnia or excessive sleepiness, that affect a person's ability to function during the day.

- **Smoke**: A collection of airborne solid and liquid particulates and gases emitted when a substance undergoes combustion. Smoke inhalation can be harmful to health.
- **Snake Plants**: A type of indoor plant known for its air-purifying qualities and low maintenance. It is believed to improve indoor air quality by removing toxins.
- **Spider Plants**: Another popular indoor plant known for its air-cleaning properties and ability to thrive in indirect sunlight.
- **Stored Fuels and Automotive Products**: Items such as gasoline, diesel, oil, and other chemicals stored for use in vehicles or machinery. Improper storage can lead to fire hazards or toxic exposure.
- **Storms**: Severe weather conditions involving strong winds, rain, thunder, or lightning, which can cause damage to property and pose safety risks.
- **Stress**: A state of mental or emotional strain resulting from adverse or demanding circumstances, which can affect overall health and well-being.
- **Strokes**: A medical condition where poor blood flow to the brain results in cell death, causing physical and cognitive impairments.
- **Sustainable Activities**: Actions and practices aimed at meeting present needs without compromising the ability of future generations to meet their needs, such as recycling or conserving energy.
- **Swimming Pools**: Man-made bodies of water used for recreational or competitive swimming, which require

proper safety measures like self-closing gates and water quality management.

- **Tablets**: Portable electronic devices with a touchscreen interface, used for various applications such as reading, browsing, and entertainment.
- **Television Commercials**: Advertisements broadcasted on television, designed to promote products, services, or ideas to a broad audience.
- **Television Signals**: Electronic signals transmitted to broadcast video and audio content to television sets.
- **Teratogenic Effects**: Harmful effects caused by exposure to certain substances during pregnancy, leading to developmental abnormalities or birth defects.
- **Threats**: Potential dangers or risks that can cause harm or damage to people, property, or the environment.
- **Throat Irritation**: Discomfort or inflammation in the throat, often caused by infections, allergens, or pollutants.
- **Toxic**: Refers to substances that are harmful or poisonous to living organisms. Toxicity depends on the dose and exposure duration.
- **Toxic Pollutants**: Harmful chemicals or materials released into the environment that can cause adverse effects on human health and ecosystems.
- **Toxicity Level**: The degree to which a substance can cause harm to an organism. This varies depending on concentration and exposure duration.

- **Traps**: Devices designed to catch or hold animals, pests, or other objects. They are used for controlling pests or for safety purposes.
- **Tree Roots**: The underground part of a tree that absorbs water and nutrients and anchors the tree to the ground. They can cause tripping hazards or damage to infrastructure.
- **Tripping Hazards**: Objects or conditions that could cause a person to trip and fall, such as uneven surfaces, cords, or clutter.
- **Trypanosome**: A genus of parasitic protozoa that cause diseases such as African sleeping sickness and Chagas disease in humans and animals.
- **Tuberculosis**: A contagious bacterial infection caused by *Mycobacterium tuberculosis*, affecting mainly the lungs but can spread to other organs.
- **Tularemia**: A rare infectious disease caused by the *Francisella tularensis* bacterium, typically spread through contact with infected animals or contaminated water.
- **Typhoid**: An infectious disease caused by the bacterium *Salmonella typhi*, usually spread through contaminated food and water, leading to fever, weakness, and abdominal pain.
- **Uneven Surfaces**: Irregular or rough surfaces that can cause tripping or falling accidents, commonly found in outdoor or poorly maintained areas.
- **Unhygienic Conditions**: Environments that lack cleanliness and sanitation, increasing the risk of disease transmission and health hazards.

- **Uranium**: A naturally occurring radioactive element used as fuel in nuclear power plants and for military purposes. Exposure to uranium can pose significant health risks.
- **Ventilation**: The process of exchanging or circulating air in a space to remove pollutants, moisture, and odors, improving indoor air quality.
- **Viral Infections**: Illnesses caused by viruses, which can affect various parts of the body and range from mild to severe.
- **Viruses**: Microscopic infectious agents that replicate inside living host cells, causing diseases in humans, animals, and plants.
- **VOCs (Volatile Organic Compounds)**: Organic chemicals that evaporate easily at room temperature, found in many household products, and can cause health problems like respiratory issues.
- **Vomiting**: The forceful expulsion of stomach contents through the mouth, often due to illness, poisoning, or other medical conditions.
- **Washing Machines**: Household appliances used for cleaning clothes and textiles. They need proper maintenance to prevent mold and bacterial growth.
- **Western Equine**: Refers to Western equine encephalitis, a viral disease transmitted by mosquitoes that can cause brain inflammation in humans and horses.
- **Wood Chips**: Small pieces of wood often used as mulch in gardening or landscaping. They help retain soil moisture and suppress weeds.

- **Wood Preservatives**: Chemicals applied to wood to protect it from decay, pests, and weathering. Some can be toxic and require careful handling.
- **World Health Organization (WHO)**: A specialized agency of the United Nations responsible for international public health, providing leadership on global health issues.
- **Zika Virus**: A mosquito-borne virus that can cause mild symptoms in adults but is linked to severe birth defects when contracted during pregnancy.

INDEX

www.ingramcontent.com/pod-product-compliance
Lightning Source LLC
LaVergne TN
LVHW052325200926
848481LV00002B/674

* 9 7 9 8 3 4 9 2 4 4 4 7 6 *

I ONLY PAINT IN WATERCOLORS

CHANGING THE LANDSCAPE

A RELATIONSHIP WITH SELF

BY NANCY ZANICCHI-BOBB

COUNSELING PSYCHOLOGY

Published by Starry Night Publishing.Com

Rochester, New York